The Vitamin Strategy

The
Vitamin Strategy

Art Ulene, MD
Val Ulene, MD

Ulysses Press

Published by: Ulysses Press
                P.O. Box 3440
                Berkeley, CA 94703-3440

ISBN: 0-915233-94-0

Printed in the USA

Editor: Barbara Fuller
Cover Design: Bonnie Smetts Design
Editorial and production staff: Ellen Nidy, Jennifer Wilkoff, Per Casey
Indexer: Sayre Van Young
Background photography: Roger Rosenfeld; authors' photo: David Quinney
Color separation: Twin Age Limited, Hong Kong

Distributed in the United States by Publishers Group West,
in Canada by Raincoast Books, and in Great Britain and Europe by World
Leisure Marketing.

Acknowledgements

The authors gratefully acknowledge:

- The scientific advice we received from Jeffrey Blumberg, PhD, FACN, Professor of Nutrition, Tufts University.

- The skillful writing and tireless work of Richard Trubo.

- The expertise and diligence of the editor Barbara Fuller.

- The guidance, talent, and tenacity of Kukla Vera.

- The competent and endless administrative support of Jamie McDowell.

CONTENTS

A Message from Dr. Art Ulene

I was wrong about vitamins.

Twenty years ago, I told my television viewers that most people didn't need vitamin supplements. If you were eating well, I said, buying and consuming vitamin pills was a waste of money.

I certainly wasn't alone in this belief. At the time, few people in the medical community supported vitamin supplementation. Even today, most physicians, and perhaps most registered dietitians and nutritionists, insist that people in the United States get all the vitamins they need from their diet alone. It's not surprising that health professionals feel this way. After all, that's what we were taught in school.

Many years ago, however, a wise professor told me, "Fifty percent of what you'll learn in medical school will later be proven wrong." (Unfortunately, he couldn't tell me which 50 percent, or I could have spared myself a lot of anguish.) I now know that many of the pronouncements I heard about the uselessness of vitamins simply aren't true. No matter what your age, no matter what your health status, according to new research, optimal doses of vitamins and minerals can improve the state of your health and reduce your chances of developing many diseases and disorders once considered to be almost unavoidable.

For years, I preached a different sermon. With the best of intentions, I gave advice that I would not offer today. Why the difference in my thinking? Our knowledge relating to nutritional supplementation has changed—at least for several specific nutrients. And this new knowledge requires all of us to reconsider our attitudes and amend the advice we give in this area. It has pointed me in a dramatically different direction, moving me to advocate an individualized vitamin and mineral supplementation program for virtually everyone.

In this book, we'll show you the evidence that has compelled me to change my mind about vitamin and mineral supplements—and that may change your way of thinking, too. We describe studies that have reached some rather remarkable conclusions about optimal vitamin intakes. We explain research that proves—at least for some nutrients—that diet alone cannot provide you with ideal levels. You'll find not only the general information that all of us need to know about vitamins and minerals, but also the strategies to create a personalized nutrition program appropriate for your unique needs.

Our knowledge is not yet complete. We now believe that some vitamins may provide protection against certain types of cancer, but we are not sure how this occurs, or precisely how much of each vitamin is necessary to give you this protection. We believe that certain vitamins may enhance the way the immune system functions, but we don't yet know the ideal vitamin combination and doses necessary to achieve this result.

Even so, our evolving and growing body of research has led to a shift in paradigm regarding supplemental vitamins and minerals. Many people have changed their thinking about who needs supplements and how much they need. These people no longer believe that we can rely solely on diet to meet our vitamin and mineral requirements. In some cases (vitamin E, for example), you clearly *cannot* get the optimal amount of a vitamin from dietary sources alone. Even for those vitamins that you *could* get strictly through diet, government surveys show that most people simply don't. In this hectic era, when so many of us eat our meals on the run, people don't have time to prepare and eat the well-balanced, varied diets that could help them meet their vitamin and mineral needs.

Bear in mind, however, that we do not recommend in this book that you take nutrient *supplements* as nutrient *substitutes*. We do not encourage you to dismiss or disregard health-promoting behaviors like reducing the fat in your diet, increasing your fiber intake, or quitting cigarette smoking. We do, however, provide you with an additional proactive method—specifically the use of diet and, if necessary, supplements—to provide you with optimal doses of nutrients crucial to your health.

I hope this book will inspire you to look more carefully at your nutritional patterns, and to make whatever changes are necessary to optimize your intake of vitamins and minerals. When you do that, you will be taking a big step on the path toward optimal health and well-being.

—Art Ulene, M.D.

A Message from Dr. Val Ulene

Despite my father's skepticism about supplemental vitamins for many years, I grew up taking vitamin tablets daily. At the time, I didn't care why my mother required me and my brothers to take the chewable tablets. After all, they contained a little sugar, and when things tasted that good, I knew better than to raise questions about them.

Eventually, however, I outgrew the chewable supplements and entered the impossible period called adolescence—when I gave up on vitamins altogether. At the same time, my dietary habits in general took a turn for the worse. I skipped meals—lots of them. And when I did eat, my diet much too often consisted only of junk food. I developed a distaste for milk and gave up fruit juice in exchange for diet soda. Rather than rely on nutritious sack lunches, I turned to a parade of rather unhealthful food purchased throughout the day.

My dietary habits hardly improved in college. In the dormitory cafeteria, dessert was always the first item in the food line. Often I ate my meals in reverse order. Many times, when the dessert was particularly good, I never quite got to the main course at all. Yes, the subject of vitamin supplements did arise from time to time in conversations with my friends, but there always seemed to be something else to spend my money on.

Not until medical school did I finally become aware that my dietary negligence might be having ill effects on my body. In physiology, I learned that our bones stop growing when we're in our 20s. In pathology, I saw slides of blood vessels clogged with cholesterol plaques. (These were particularly frightening because they were the arteries of 20- and 30-year-olds.)

Disease, I discovered, does not happen suddenly in old age. It's a dynamic process that begins years (often decades) before symptoms appear. I also learned that many diseases—from osteoporosis to atherosclerosis—are not inevitable, as I had once believed them to be; they can be prevented, often through changes in diet.

The more I studied and the more I learned, the more I began to appreciate the importance of proper nutrition. I made some major improvements in my diet. I recognized, however, that those adjustments wouldn't be enough. As conscientious as I tried to be, I realized, my fast-paced lifestyle made it virtually impossible for me to eat properly all the time. To complicate matters, scientific literature suggested that even a perfect diet wouldn't supply optimal amounts of all the vitamins and minerals I need.

That's when I decided to make supplements part of my daily routine. I started taking a multivitamin daily, as well as individual daily doses of vitamins C and E, beta-carotene, calcium, and iron. And the more I learned about these supplements, the more conscientious I became about taking them—every day.

The vitamin and mineral tablets I take now do not taste as good as the chewable ones from my childhood, but more compelling reasons keep me taking vitamins these days. As you will read in this book, a carefully designed, personalized program of vitamin and mineral supplementation can help each of us achieve optimal health. In the weeks and months ahead, I hope you will use this information to take some giant strides toward becoming as healthy as you can possibly be.

—Val Ulene, M.D.

INTRODUCTION

We live in an age of medical miracles. Procedures like bone marrow transplants and coronary bypass surgery are now being used to save lives that would have been lost a generation ago. These kinds of headline-grabbing technological breakthroughs are revolutionizing the way medicine is practiced today.

At the same time, a gentler—but no less important—revolution is taking place in the field of nutrition. Knowledge and attitudes about vitamins and minerals are changing dramatically. So, too, is the way we are using these important nutrients.

Until recently, vitamins and minerals were considered important primarily for avoiding deficiency-related medical disorders. Consume enough vitamin C, we were told, to prevent scurvy. Take just enough iron and folic acid, we were advised, to prevent anemia. And so on for each nutrient: vitamin A to prevent night blindness, vitamin D to prevent rickets, thiamin to prevent beriberi. Medical and nutritional experts recommended doses of each vitamin and mineral at a level just high enough to ward off these deficiency diseases.

But recent research has transformed the way we look at these nutrients and caused many authorities to alter their recommendations for intake levels. New studies have demonstrated that certain vitamins and minerals may do much more than prevent deficiency disorders—especially when taken in large amounts. Evidence indicates that higher levels of selected nutrients may actually slow or prevent the physical deterioration associated with aging—a deterioration once considered to be inevitable. Indeed, proper supplements of vitamins and minerals may help many people prevent some of the most common chronic diseases and illnesses associated with aging—from heart disease and cancer to cataracts.

This nutritional approach is part of an entirely new way of looking at aging and health. In the past, we've assumed that our health would decline as we grew older and that the frequency, severity, and duration of our illnesses and disorders would increase. Today, many physicians believe that we can significantly retard the process of aging by changing the way we eat, increasing our physical activity levels, avoiding cigarettes, limiting alcohol intake, and—yes—taking supplements of certain vitamins and minerals.

The goal of this approach is not merely to prevent disease, but to attain optimal health, or high-level wellness. The idea is that, instead of spending our early years in good health and our later years in physical decline, we'll be able to live our entire lives in good health—right up to the day we die.

Will vitamin and mineral supplements alone enable us to accomplish this goal? No. But there is now good reason to believe that such supplements—in combination with a healthy lifestyle—can significantly contribute toward our achieving this goal.

Despite growing evidence about the importance of vitamins and minerals, however, most people in the United States still know little about these nutrients. Even with all the information about nutrition now available in magazines and newspapers and on television and radio, few people are familiar with the Recommended Dietary Allowances (RDAs) for vitamins and minerals. According to one survey, for example, while many people know that oranges are a good source of vitamin C, these people don't know how many oranges it takes to meet the RDA for vitamin C. Nor can they describe the kinds and quantities of other foods that could help them meet the RDA for this vitamin—or for any other vitamin or mineral.

About 35 percent of the people surveyed described themselves as regular users of nutritional supplements (meaning that they took vitamin and mineral supplements on a daily or near-daily basis). The majority of these people took supplements as "cheap insurance" against nutritional deficiencies. (Many recognized that they were not eating well-balanced diets.) Some believed that the extra nutrients could enhance their levels of health and wellness.

In our own informal survey of supplement users, we found a small (but, we think, rapidly growing) group of people who took nutritional supplements because their doctors had recommended that they do so. Most of these people had been advised to take a multivitamin and mineral preparation that contained no more than the RDA for any particular nutrient.

When we asked regular supplement users how they decided which specific vitamins and minerals to take—and in what quantities— most said they merely guessed which preparations and doses would be best for them or selected brands they learned about through advertising. Others took the advice of store clerks or friends or relied on magazine articles. A few followed the recommendations of their doctor or pharmacist. Most of these people complained of confusion over the many nutritional products available in stores today.

What about the majority of people in the United States, who do not classify themselves as regular users of nutritional supplements? Some we interviewed said they took an occasional dose of one or more vitamins or minerals. But most chose not to take any supplements because they believed they could get all of the nutrients they needed in their diets. Several indicated that they *would* use nutritional supplements if their doctors told them it was important to do so—but that hadn't happened.

In fact, the diets of most people in this country do not include even the *minimum* amounts of vitamins and minerals recommended to avoid deficiency problems. Although the United States is the richest nation on Earth, with healthful foods widely available in our supermarkets, government surveys show that most people here do not consume the RDAs. If "you are what you eat," it's no wonder that our doctors' offices and hospitals are filled with people whose illnesses might have been prevented or forestalled by better nutrition.

A note of caution is in order. As important as increased doses of particular nutrients may be, excessive amounts of some—for example, preformed vitamin A, vitamin B$_6$, and iron—can produce serious toxic side effects and even permanent physical damage. It's important to be prudent and cautious in using vitamin and mineral supplements, then, and always to try to maximize the benefits while minimizing the risks. We'll show you how to do that in the pages that follow.

The bottom line? It's time to question the old conventional wisdom about vitamin and mineral supplements. Optimal well-being is more than just absence of disease; it is a state of exuberant wellness and of efficient, effortless function. If optimal health is your goal, this book will help you reach that goal.

THE VITAMIN STRATEGY

In your efforts to stay healthy throughout your life, you will find that vitamins and minerals can be significantly more potent than you might now realize. *The Vitamin Strategy* will show you how to make the most of these nutrients in your diet and how to determine when supplements are appropriate and which ones to take in what quantities. We have created our vitamin and mineral strategy with the intention that you adapt it as a part of your own health-promoting lifestyle.

Developing Your Own Vitamin and Mineral Strategy

Although only 35 percent of the people in the United States classify themselves as regular vitamin takers, in truth, we are *all* vitamin takers. Some of us rely exclusively on the foods we eat for our vitamins; others consider supplements important. Some consume less of the essential nutrients than we need; others take far more than necessary.

So how do you create your own strategy? Do you take the word of government scientists and adhere to Recommended Dietary Allowances (which are revised about every five years and will certainly be changed again)? Do you follow the advice of the clerk at the health food store (who may earn a commission on the sale of certain products)? Is it sufficient simply to eat a "balanced" diet (whatever that means), or should you supplement your diet with vitamin and mineral pills? And if you do use supplements, how do you know what amounts to take?

The answers to these questions are not simple. However, as we spoke to nutrition researchers across the nation while putting together this book, it became clear that you do not have to wait years to get the information necessary for making prudent decisions about vitamins and minerals. In fact, enough research has been compiled on many vitamins and minerals for you to make thoughtful, knowledgeable, and safe choices about individual nutrients.

Using the information in this book, you can create your own vitamin and mineral strategy. In the pages that follow, we put science on your side and show you how to use the existing research—along with your own good judgment—to determine what nutrients you should take, and in what quantities.

Meeting Your Nutritional Needs

One of the unique aspects of *The Vitamin Strategy* is its personalized nature. This book will show you how to determine your own nutritional needs and how best to meet them. Toward that goal, you need to know the answers to the following questions:

How much of each vitamin and mineral do you need to consume in order to achieve optimal health? This book includes profiles of each of the major vitamins and minerals. As part of our description of each nutrient, we include a section titled "Optimal Daily Allowance." Here you'll find our careful determination as to how much of the nutrient you should take—in your diet, through supplements, or both—for the healthiest life possible.

For some vitamins and minerals, we make a single recommendation for everyone—a target dose of niacin or vitamin B_6, for example, that will meet your needs, whether you are in good health or you have minor or even serious health problems. For other nutrients, we provide a recommended dosage range. You select which part of the scale is most appropriate for you, based on your age, sex, and medical conditions.

Do special circumstances in your life affect the amount of a particular vitamin or mineral you need to maintain optimal health? To answer this question, refer to the section in each chapter titled, "Who's at Risk?" Certain factors may interfere with your body's ability to absorb and utilize specific vitamins. Some people, for example, have trouble digesting milk products, which are a rich source of calcium, vitamin D, and other nutrients. Or an intestinal disorder could interfere with your ability to absorb fat-soluble vitamins (A, D, E, and K), so you may need more of these vitamins to make up for the amount that's not absorbed. Cigarette smokers require at least twice as much vitamin C as nonsmokers. And so on. When we provide you with a recommended dosage range for a given vitamin, use this risk-related information to help find your personal optimal consumption level.

In cases where we recommend a single dose, that level is high enough to compensate for increased risks based on lifestyle or on any illnesses you may have. The single recommended dose will not only prevent deficiencies and make up for special medical conditions, but also help you attain an optimal level of health.

Can you consume the optimal amount of a given vitamin or mineral through diet alone? We help you answer this question with a self-test in each vitamin and mineral chapter. To evaluate the foods you eat on a typical day, use the section called, "How Much Are You Getting?"

You may be able to meet your needs for certain vitamins and minerals easily through diet alone. The RDA and our own recommended optimal dose of vitamin A, for instance, are both 1,000 mcg of RE (retinol equivalents), or 5,000 IU. A one-cup serving of cantaloupe pieces contains 516 mcg of vitamin A, meeting about half of your total needs for the day. A single medium-sized carrot (2,025 mcg) or one sweet potato (2,488 mcg) provides more than the optimal amount. In addition to our recommendation for vitamin A, we make a separate daily recommendation for beta-carotene, an important antioxidant and a precursor of vitamin A. That recommendation ranges from 6 mg per day to 30 mg, depending on the individual. Here again, a carrot or two can meet the needs of many people. So for some of the nutrients you read about in this book, you can reach your optimal daily requirements simply by making wise food choices.

The task, however, is not so simple for a nutrient such as vitamin E—especially if you share our belief that, ideally, you should take several times more of this important vitamin than the government's guidelines suggest. Although the Recommended Dietary Allowance of vitamin E is 30 IU per day, we believe that all adults should get at least 100 IU per day—and some should have as much as 400 IU. To reach the RDA, you'd have to eat 60 medium-sized apricots, or nearly 100 dried prunes per day! To meet the high end (400 IU) of our optimal recommendation, you'd need to consume even larger quantities of food—400 apricots, about 650 prunes, or a combination of these or similar foods—each day. That's just not practical.

In sections titled "Health Merits," you will find descriptions of the cutting-edge research on which we base many of our optimal-dose recommendations. Recent studies have clearly proven the value of supplemental folic acid in preventing birth defects, for example. As a result, most experts now agree that every woman of child-bearing age should take extra folic acid *before* becoming pregnant and throughout her entire pregnancy. This is the kind of information you need to personalize your vitamin strategy.

Equally persuasive data can help you make decisions about other vitamins and minerals. Recent research has revealed a dramatically reduced risk of heart attack among men and women who have supplemented their diets with vitamin E, for example—but only if they have taken at least 100 IU of vitamin E per day for at least two-and-a-half years.

So how much vitamin E should you take? Based on this research, you could argue that 100 IU per day is enough. But you could also make a good case for taking up to 400 IU per day if you were a large person, if you had a strong history of heart disease in your family, or if you were at high risk for a heart attack because of high blood cholesterol levels or other factors.

The Rationale for the Vitamin Strategy

As you adapt our vitamin strategy to your needs, keep in mind the following underlying principles we used in designing it.

Strategy 1: The goal of vitamin and mineral intake is not just to prevent deficiency diseases, but to help your body achieve a state of optimal health. Set your nutrient doses at a level designed to produce maximum well-being rather than simply to avoid symptoms associated with deficiencies.

For decades—and even today—most vitamin and mineral recommendations have been based on the lowest level necessary to prevent deficiency symptoms, with a modest margin of safety added. The scientific panel that sets RDAs recently stated that its recommendations are for "the levels of intake of essential nutrients that, on the basis of scientific knowledge, are judged by the Food and Nutrition Board to be adequate to meet the known nutrient needs of practically all healthy persons." The panel stated that it was impossible to determine and establish "optimal" doses higher than the RDAs.

We strongly disagree with this approach and philosophy. First, many people are not "healthy" (a term defined differently by just about everyone anyway). The RDA level may be much too low for people who have medical disorders such as diabetes or kidney disease, who use alcohol or certain medications, or who have unusual dietary patterns. Some of these individuals should take many times the RDA of specific nutrients to compensate for their circumstances.

Also, despite what RDA panelists have said, strong evidence now suggests that larger doses of at least some nutrients can do far more than simply prevent deficiency diseases. Increased amounts of selected vitamins and minerals may help prevent some of the conditions of aging once considered inevitable (we discuss many specific examples in later chapters). To the extent that you can potentially benefit from larger doses, it makes sense to us to increase doses—provided the monetary cost is reasonable and the potential risk of adverse reactions is low. We believe most people should take more of many vitamins and minerals than the RDAs.

Strategy 2: For each nutrient, the optimal dose should provide the best balance of benefits with the least potential risk. As with most things in life, the goal of nutritional planning is to gain the greatest possible good without putting yourself in jeopardy. Whenever potential benefits of higher vitamin levels outweigh potential risks, taking the vitamins makes sense.

Unfortunately, the situation is not always clear-cut. At low doses, benefits do generally outweigh risks. But for most vitamins and minerals, few statistically sound studies have accurately measured the risks and benefits at higher intake levels. Medical literature is, however, filled with reports of dangerous side effects at extremely high doses for some nutrients. We describe these dangers in individual vitamin and mineral chapters.

Because many physicians and nutritional experts fear adverse effects, they continue to advise that everyone take only the relatively conservative RDA levels for all vitamins and minerals. We think differently on this matter. We agree that levels at or near the RDAs make sense for selected nutrients whose toxic levels can be reached fairly quickly, particularly when no clear evidence indicates that larger doses offer additional health benefits. But we also believe the reverse. For vitamin E, for example, research strongly suggests major benefits from larger doses, and no significant side effects have been found among people who have taken increased doses for long periods of time. It makes sense, we think, to boost the amount of vitamin E you take to the range we recommend.

If a situation is unclear, we believe the prudent course generally is to take the lower doses until evidence indicates either that higher levels are risk-free or that higher levels confer sufficient additional benefits to warrant some risks. We help you make these decisions throughout this book.

Strategy 3: When appropriate, personalize your strategy to meet your unique needs in terms of age, sex, size, lifestyle, and medical condition. In the individual vitamin and mineral chapters, we guide you in deciding if you require extra quantities of a particular nutrient because of your unique circumstances. Do you need additional iron because you are a woman whose menstrual periods are especially heavy? If so, you should consider this in finding your place within the range we advise. For other vitamins and minerals, a single recommended dose is appropriate for everyone, making up for deficiencies and shortcomings and promoting optimal health.

Strategy 4: Use foods as your source of vitamins and minerals whenever possible. In this regard, we agree with the traditionalists who criticize the use of nutritional supplements. Through a varied and balanced diet, you can provide your body with a variety of the vitamins and minerals you need, without risks of side effects. Keep in mind, too, that foods supply you with other important substances that you can't get from a vitamin pill, from energy-producing proteins and carbohydrates to cholesterol-lowering fibers.

However, you may not be able to get enough of the necessary nutrients through foods alone. If you're on a low-calorie diet for weight loss, if your body does not tolerate dairy products, or if a chronic disease interferes with your absorption of nutrients, for example, you will need to supplement your meals with vitamin and mineral pills.

Strategy 5: Use vitamins and minerals to complement a healthful lifestyle—not to compensate for unhealthful habits. Some people believe they can make up for all kinds of undesirable behaviors by taking vitamin and mineral supplements. But a vitamin pill certainly can't replace the cardiovascular and many other benefits of exercise. And while vitamins may help overcome free-radical formation stimulated by cigarette smoking, they won't protect you from nicotine's destructive effects upon your heart. In the same way, if you eat a lot of high-fat foods or have other unhealthful habits, a few vitamin and mineral capsules won't rescue you from a health crisis at some point in your life. Nutritional supplements should be an adjunct to the other health-enhancing behaviors that are part of your day-to-day living.

Using This Book

With these strategies as its base, this book will show you what each nutrient does and how it works. You will also learn whether you are more likely than most to develop nutrient deficiencies and therefore need larger doses of particular vitamins and minerals.

For each nutrient, we give the RDA. But just as significantly—or perhaps more so—we introduce you to our recommended doses (Optimal Daily Allowances) and show you how we arrived at them. Then, at the end of each vitamin and mineral chapter, we summarize the most critical information in "Our Recommendations." Here you can quickly find the optimal dose of a vitamin or mineral, the circumstances that could affect your need for it, and whether you can consume enough of it through diet alone.

On page 258 you will find "The Vitamin Planner," an easy-to-use chart to record your vitamin and mineral intake obtained through your diet, and the amount needed from supplements in order to reach your Optimal Daily Allowance. Be sure to talk over with your physician any medical disorders you may have, particularly in terms of the nutrient adjustments we recommend because of them.

On the illness-to-wellness continuum, we'd like to see you move as far to the wellness end of the spectrum as possible. If you use the information in this book to create a vitamin and mineral strategy for yourself, we believe, you may be within closer reach of optimal health than you have ever been before.

THE FACTS ABOUT VITAMINS AND MINERALS

With all the current interest in vitamins and minerals, nearly everyone is getting the message that these nutrients are important to our health and well-being. But many people don't really understand what vitamins and minerals are, why they're so crucial, and how to go about buying them. This chapter is designed to provide this kind of information.

Vitamin and Mineral Basics

Let's begin with vitamins: organic (carbon-containing) substances derived from living material (animals or plants) and essential in small amounts for good health. We currently know about 13 vitamins. These play many critical roles in the body; among other things, they promote proper vision, blood clotting, and formation of hormones and genetic material; maintain tissues; and strengthen the immune system. Vitamins are also important for the processing of other nutrients and for the functioning of the body's enzyme systems.

Your body generally needs only small amounts of vitamins. We obtain most of these nutrients through diet, with a couple of exceptions. Your skin manufactures vitamin D when exposed to sunlight, and our body produces niacin (though somewhat inefficiently) if you consume enough of an amino acid called tryptophan.

Our knowledge about vitamins is relatively recent. Scientists identified the first vitamin—now known as vitamin A—in 1913. When researchers discovered that the chemical structure of this nutrient contained an *amine* (a nitrogen-containing chemical compound), they labeled the important substance *vitamine* (an amine vital to life). The e was eventually dropped from the name, and these nutrients have since been referred to as *vitamins*.

Vitamins constitute one of several categories of nutrients necessary for normal body growth, maintenance, and tissue repair. Some nutrients—fats, carbohydrates, and proteins—are referred to as *macronutrients;* they make up most of our diet and supply the body with energy. Others—vitamins and minerals—are *micronutrients;* they are a relatively small part of our diet and are not a source of energy (though some vitamins help convert calorie-containing nutrients into usable forms of energy). Even so, micronutrients are as essential to good health as their macro counterparts, and most foods contain both.

What about minerals? Although vitamins have received much more attention, minerals are just as important. While vitamins are *organic* substances (containing carbon), minerals are *inorganic* substances (not bound to carbon). Minerals originate in soil and water but find their way into the animals and plants that make up our diet. Minerals play many crucial roles in the proper functioning of the body. Some are part of important enzyme systems necessary for biochemical reactions to occur. Some help keep the heart beating properly; others make sure that oxygen gets to every cell in the body. Minerals help build strong bones and teeth and are necessary for the manufacture of hemoglobin, the oxygen-carrying portion of the blood.

Your body needs much larger quantities of many minerals than of vitamins. Each day, we need hundreds of milligrams of the minerals called *macro* (or *major*) minerals, which include calcium, sodium, potassium, chloride, phosphorus, sulfur, and magnesium. Your body requires only small amounts of other minerals, called *trace* minerals, including iron, iodine, and copper. Relatively little is known about other trace minerals—nickel, tin, and vanadium—but researchers believe that they are probably necessary at very small levels. No mineral is more crucial than others; your body needs all of them in appropriate quantities.

FAT-SOLUBLE OR WATER-SOLUBLE?

All vitamins are either fat-soluble or water-soluble. These categories help define absorption, storage, and other characteristics of nutrients.

Fat-soluble vitamins are A, D, E, and K. As their name suggests, these vitamins dissolve in liquid fats but not in water. The body absorbs them through the intestinal tract membranes with the assistance of dietary fats and bile acids. Once absorbed, these vitamins are transported and stored throughout the body; in many cases the body can call upon these reserves if intake of a vitamin is low. Because these nutrients can accumulate in the body, toxic levels of vitamin A, D, and K in particular occur relatively quickly with consistently high consumption levels.

Water-soluble vitamins are C and all of the Bs. The body absorbs these vitamins through the gastrointestinal tract—without the help of dietary fats and bile acids—and does not store significant amounts of them. Because excess quantities are excreted (lost through urination or perspiration), the body is less likely to build up toxic levels of water-soluble vitamins than of fat-soluble vitamins. You need to be more conscientious about consuming adequate amounts of water-soluble vitamins on a regular basis, however. These nutrients also tend to be less sturdy than fat-soluble nutrients and are more likely to be destroyed in storage, through cooking, or when exposed to light.

HOW MUCH DO YOU NEED?

The amounts of vitamins and minerals that you need depend on your criteria for need. Are you taking nutrients simply to avoid symptoms of deficiencies? Or are you reaching for vitamin levels that optimize your health?

This book is designed to help you find your personal *optimal* dose of each vitamin and mineral. In most cases, we recommend more of a nutrient than the *Recommended Dietary Allowance*, or RDA. In general, RDAs are considered safe and adequate, but not necessarily optimal.

The RDAs were first issued in the 1940s by the Food and Nutrition Board of the National Academy of Science's National Research Council. The board periodically updates the RDAs, based on the latest research findings. Never intended as hard-and-fast requirements, the RDAs were created by nutritional scientists who calculated the body's need for each nutrient and then added a little more as a safety factor to compensate for individual variability. Not everyone is content with the RDAs, however. Many nutritional experts now believe that the recommended doses may avoid deficiencies but are not high enough to help prevent chronic diseases and promote truly optimal health.

The RDAs, listed in each of the vitamin and mineral chapters in this book, include separate recommendations for each sex, for different age categories (from infancy to old age), and for women who are pregnant or breast-feeding. In the 1970s, officials at the U.S. Food and Drug Administration (FDA) felt a need to make the RDAs simpler and more accessible, particularly for placing this information on food-packaging labels. As a result, the FDA issued its own *U.S. Recommended Daily Allowances*, or USRDAs—a single recommendation for each vitamin and mineral. In general, USRDAs correspond to the highest RDA for each nutrient. More recently, the FDA has decided to replace the USRDA with a new term, *Reference Daily Intake*, or RDI; this term is now beginning to appear on food labels. (See "Reading a Food Label," following.)

READING A FOOD LABEL

One of the best ways to assure that your diet is rich in vitamins and minerals is to purchase foods that contain high amounts of these nutrients. By reading food labels, you can discriminate in the foods you buy.

Millions of people in the United States—85 percent, according to one survey—already read food labels. Many depend on the information they get from these labels to choose the items they will place in their supermarket carts; 75 percent of consumers say they pass up products if they don't like what they read.

Despite this apparent concern for good nutrition, however, many individuals find the information on labels confusing and difficult to apply to their own diet in a useful way. While the FDA mandates that nearly all processed foods carry nutritional information, deciphering and utilizing that information has often been difficult.

This may be changing. Since May 1994, the FDA has taken some of the guesswork out of the process, thanks to its new and more accessible labeling guidelines. The list of vitamins and minerals required on many food items is now more complete. (Ironically, the new regulations no longer require listing a few vitamins—thiamin, riboflavin, and niacin—because deficiencies of these nutrients are no longer considered a significant public health problem in the United States.) The term *Reference Daily Intake (RDI)* has replaced the old USRDA.

The new labeling system introduces another new name, *Daily Reference Values (DRVs)*. These numbers provide information on specific food components—fat, saturated fat, cholesterol, sodium, fiber, carbohydrate, potassium, and protein—that have been linked with the development of (or a decrease in) various chronic diseases.

HOW TO BUY VITAMINS AND MINERALS

As you read this book, you may decide that, for the good of your health, you want to consume more vitamins and minerals than you get from your meals. That may lead you to the nutrient-supplement section of your supermarket, to a health food store, or to mail-order ads, where the wide array of available supplements may boggle you.

Don't panic. Following are some guidelines to help you navigate through the maze of vitamin and mineral choices.

NATURAL OR SYNTHETIC

As you browse the vitamin shelves, you'll face a decision between *natural* and *synthetic* supplements. Natural products come from foods, while synthetic versions are manufactured in a lab. It's a confusing issue, and many consumers believe that they cheat themselves if they "settle" for synthetic vitamins rather than paying more for natural versions.

Despite the hype, the natural and synthetic formulations of each nutrient have the same chemical configuration, whether they were obtained from plants or made in a laboratory. Once you remove them from the bottle and swallow them, they act identically; your body won't know the difference. Some "natural" products, in fact, might actually be a combination of a little bit of plant extract and synthetic vitamins; the word *natural* means whatever the manufacturer wants it to mean.

There are exceptions to this rule: the natural and synthetic formulations of vitamin E and beta-carotene have minor differences in their chemical configuration. Some people believe the natural versions have greater efficacy. Frankly, the variations may be too subtle to be significant. If you want to spend a little more on the natural product in hopes that it will be more effective, go ahead. The issue is still unresolved.

Be aware, too, that some manufacturers promote their products as originating from various sources—most commonly, vitamin C from "rose hips." In general, you do not need to be concerned about this. In fact, many "rose hip" vitamins are probably mostly synthetic, with only a small amount of the C coming from the fleshy base (the hip) of the rose itself. The rest has been manufactured in a test tube, just as any other synthetic vitamin.

In addition to the natural-synthetic debate, manufacturers of some synthetic forms of vitamins and minerals claim that their supplements are more available to the body. "Ester C" for example, may have 10 percent greater "bioavailability" than traditional vitamin C. Even a 10 percent variation, however, won't make a lot of difference when you're already consuming 250 to 500 mg of vitamin C.

WHERE TO SHOP

There's no shortage of places to buy nutritional supplements. Supermarkets sell them, as do pharmacies, health food stores, some department stores, and mail-order houses.

So where should you shop? Except for some variations in price, you may not find much difference among the supplements from one store to another. Only a limited number of companies manufacture vitamins and minerals. These supply brand-name products to outlets throughout the country and also repackage their items with store-brand labels. So while the names on the labels may change, the products are generally identical. Still, just to be safe, it's a good idea to buy supplements at a store known for selling quality merchandise.

SUPPLEMENT LABELS

As with any other product you buy, do some comparison shopping—and not only for price. Read the labels on supplements, and see what you get for your dollar. Don't allow gimmicky names—such as *stress vitamins*, *therapeutic formulas*, or *super vitamins*—to sway you. Instead, look at the description of what's inside the bottle, specifically at the nutrients and their potencies.

Using your personalized program as a guide, you need to determine, for example, if a multivitamin formulation can give you the amounts of each nutrient that you want. Would you be better off purchasing certain vitamin or mineral supplements individually? For most people, the answer is probably in combining a broad-spectrum multivitamin and mineral preparation with "booster" doses of selected individual nutrients to meet particular needs.

Be sure to look carefully at the quantities of nutrients in the bottle. Often you'll find quantities given in milligrams (mg), the equivalent of one-thousandth of a gram. Some vitamins and minerals are needed in such small amounts, however, that they are measured in micrograms (mcg), equal to one-millionth of a gram. Some—such as vitamins A, D, and E—may also be measured in international units (IU), designations of their biological activity, not of their weight. The labels of many products carrying IU values also provide equivalency doses in milligrams or micrograms.

When you consider price, keep in mind not only the number of tablets in the bottle, but also the amount of the nutrient in each tablet. Don't let the size of the bottle or of the capsules themselves deceive you; the quantity of a given vitamin or mineral in a single tablet can differ considerably.

The label may also give you clues about the capacity of the vitamin or mineral to dissolve in your digestive system and make its way into your bloodstream. Unless the product is a time-release formulation, it should dissolve in water and disintegrate (break into small pieces) within an hour. If it doesn't dissolve this way— and not all pills do—it can't work in your bloodstream. The label probably won't contain this specific information, but look for a designation that the manufacturer adheres to standards created by the US Pharmacopoeia (USP), the scientific body that sets criteria for drug composition. These guidelines require, for example, that water-soluble vitamins disintegrate in the digestive tract in no more than 30 to 45 minutes. If the label doesn't provide data about the release of the nutrients, or if it doesn't state that the product abides by USP standards, assume that it doesn't meet these guidelines. Also, feel free to call or write to the manufacturer and request information about the speed with which its products dissolve and disintegrate.

Check the expiration date on the label, and don't purchase a product with a date that has already passed. In fact, if a product is within a few months of expiring—say, within six months or less— it may have already been in the bottle for a few years and lost some of its stability and potency. Look for a product that doesn't expire for several more years.

USING SUPPLEMENTS

Many experts on vitamins and minerals say that your body can make use of supplements no matter what time of day you consume them. If you take them with meals, though, food can often improve the rate at which your intestines absorb the nutrients. We recommend that you take your vitamins and minerals at the same time each day—perhaps with breakfast or dinner—making it a habit and reducing the chances that you'll forget to take them.

Store your supplements away from direct sunlight and heat. A cool, dry place is better than the refrigerator, where moisture can undermine the nutrients' potency.

Selecting and properly utilizing vitamin and mineral supplements takes effort. With care, though, you can maximize the benefits you get from these nutrients and place yourself on the fast track toward optimal health.

ANTIOXIDANTS

Antioxidants Role in Optimizing Health

The dramatic change in attitude about vitamins is largely the result of impressive evidence about the group of nutrients known as antioxidants—vitamins C and E as well as beta-carotene, a compound that the body converts into vitamin A. In recent years, scientific journals have published studies, conducted at some of the world's most respected medical research facilities, supporting the role of these unique nutrients in preventing major chronic diseases and illnesses, from cancers to heart disease to cataracts.

What makes antioxidants so important? Can they really help us move from ordinary to optimal health? In this chapter, we look closely at how antioxidants work in our body, and at how consuming them can improve our health.

How Do Antioxidants Work?

To understand how antioxidants can help you, step back for a moment to look at your body as a whole and at how it functions in your environment.

Your body is a complex structure with several dynamic organ systems that function independently and interdependently. To sustain you in your environment, these interconnected systems require fuel. That fuel—the food you take in when you eat—is broken down into macronutrients: fats, carbohydrates, and proteins. Macronutrients provide the energy that enables your lungs to take in air and your heart to continuously pump blood through your body. This energy allows your brain to function, your muscles to contract, and your immune system to fight off infection.

Your body's process of consuming and using energy is called its *metabolism*. This process goes on constantly, day and night, within your body. In a way, this use of energy is like a car's burning of gasoline. The car requires the right octane of gasoline to run at full efficiency. Your body requires the right balance of macronutrients to run at its best.

The Role of Oxygen

Without oxygen, your body could not convert the food that you consume into usable energy. This essential ingredient allows you to metabolize available fats, proteins, and carbohydrates.

The body's use of oxygen involves a process known as *oxidative reactions*. These essential reactions convert energy into useful molecular subunits and discard what is no longer needed or functional.

Everything you do—from the most basic actions of seeing, hearing, smelling, and tasting to the more complex activities of walking, running, laughing, sleeping, and thinking—depends on your body's use of oxygen. Oxygen is key to your survival and to the proper functioning of your vital organs.

Free Radicals

In a car, the running motor creates an exhaust that is emitted through the tailpipe. The gases in that exhaust (carbon monoxide, sulfur, and nitrogen oxides) are harmful pollutants. In a similar way, as your body uses molecules to create energy, it produces an "exhaust" that includes substances known as free radicals. Because of their structure, free radicals are toxic; you can think of them as harmful pollutants. Of the many kinds of free radicals, the most common are oxygen-free radicals. As the cells in your body consume millions of oxygen molecules each minute, huge numbers of these oxygen-free radicals are produced.

Free radicals are molecules with one or more unpaired electrons; they are unstable and highly reactive. To regain stability, free radicals attack other molecules in search of an electron. Indeed, free radicals can target molecules in any cell in the body from which to grab an electron. The molecule attacked by the free radical loses an electron and is damaged.

Just as your body constantly consumes and uses energy, the free radicals produced during this process constantly damage molecules in cells throughout your body. In fact, every cell in your body is subjected to an estimated 10,000 "hits" by free radicals each day.

While normal metabolism produces some free radicals, many circumstances—such as illness, cigarette smoking, radiation, and irritating chemicals in the air—can increase the number of free radicals produced. When the level of free radicals gets too high, as in smokers, for example, the body is said to be in a state of *oxidative stress*.

Fortunately, your cells have built-in systems to repair the damage free radicals cause and your body can usually maintain a reasonable balance between the rate of damage and the rate of repair. Under conditions of oxidative stress, however, more time may be required to repair a cell or one of its parts. During this "catch-up" period, the damaged cell or the organ of which it is a part may still function, but at a less-than-optimal level. The cell and the organ may not be damaged enough to be considered "sick," but they certainly are not well.

Consider, for example, the oxidative damage and repair that takes place in your body if you exercise too vigorously. The working muscles consume large quantities of oxygen and produce huge numbers of free radicals. The next day, you feel muscle fatigue, largely the effect of free radical damage. If you rest for a day or two, your muscles repair themselves and the pain goes away. This is the process of oxidative stress and cellular healing.

On the other hand, the damage from free radicals is sometimes too extensive to repair. If free radicals attack and damage enough molecules, cell death may occur, and entire organs may be damaged and even cease to work, or your body's DNA molecules may be permanently damaged, which could eventually trigger the development of a disease such as cancer. Some scientists believe that free radicals are responsible for or contribute significantly to the development of a number of chronic illnesses and to aging itself.

If free radicals are so bad, you may wonder, why does your body continue to produce them? Like oxygen itself—which is essential but which can be toxic—free radicals help protect your body in some important ways. Certain immune cells in your body release free radicals that can kill invading bacteria and help prevent infection, for example. Because of this, we need to balance the destructive and the beneficial capabilities of these molecules. In most cases, fortunately, you can maintain this balance through cellular repair systems and through *antioxidants*, substances that "neutralize" free radicals before enough of them accumulate to damage the healthy cells in your body.

Antioxidant Vitamins

The substances that neutralize free radicals are called antioxidants. Some antioxidants occur naturally in the environment; your body manufactures others (for example, enzymes with names like *superoxide dismutase, glutathione peroxidase,* and *catalase*). Certain vitamins and minerals have antioxidant effects, particularly vitamins C and E, beta-carotene, zinc, and selenium. (See individual chapters for more about these micronutrients.)

Currently, our knowledge is greatest about the antioxidant effects of vitamins C and E and of beta-carotene. These three micronutrients are found in different parts of the cell; which nutrient is active depends on where a free radical attacks. For example, vitamin E is fat-soluble (dissolves in fat) and is found primarily in cell membranes; it may act most prominently as an antioxidant if damage occurs in the cell membrane. The water-soluble vitamin C is found in the cytoplasm of the cell and may play a more important antioxidant role if a free radical is inside the watery confines of the cell.

Despite their different locations in the cell, antioxidants operate in similar ways. When they encounter a free radical, with its unpaired or missing electron, they give up one of their own electrons to the free radical. Once its electron is paired, the free radical is "quenched": that is, it is no longer reactive or toxic.

Why doesn't the vitamin itself become a free radical? It does, in fact, but its structure is much more stable, so it is neither toxic nor reactive. Interestingly, antioxidants have been found to interact with each other. When vitamin E gives up its electron to a free radical, the vitamin becomes oxidized. Vitamin C can then interact with the modified vitamin E and return it to its original state. This vitamin interaction helps maintain the balance between free radicals and antioxidants.

In summation, our body breaks down the food that we consume into the nutrients that supply energy. This energy fuels the many cellular functions necessary to sustain life. Metabolism—the process of energy consumption and utilization—involves a series of reactions using oxygen. These oxidative reactions create by-products, known as free radicals, which are highly reactive, toxic molecules with unpaired electrons. In some cases, free radicals defend the body against infections; in others, they cause cellular damage. Substances known as antioxidants help the body cope with this potential for cellular damage. Antioxidants, most notably vitamins C and E and beta-carotene, give up electrons to render free radicals harmless.

Antioxidants and Chronic Diseases

As noted earlier, some scientists believe that free radicals contribute to the development of some important medical problems and chronic diseases, including cardiovascular disease (heart disease and stroke), cancer, and cataracts. To appreciate how antioxidants may prevent or delay disease, it's important to explore the role of free radicals in these areas.

CARDIOVASCULAR DISEASE DUE TO ATHEROSCLEROSIS

The primary cause of cardiovascular disease (coronary heart disease, heart attack, angina, and stroke) is a disorder called *atherosclerosis*, in which fat deposits, called *plaque*, build up in the walls of arteries. This buildup ultimately causes the openings inside the arteries to narrow, choking off the flow of blood and oxygen. If too much plaque builds up, the lack of oxygen eventually damages the organs served by the arteries. When blood flow to the heart is cut off, a heart attack occurs; when the brain is affected, a stroke results.

The process of accumulating plaque is complex and involves many factors, including elevated cholesterol levels, high blood pressure, and cigarette smoking. The level of cholesterol in the blood is important, but the action of free radicals on LDL (the so-called "bad" cholesterol) also appears to be critical. Research shows that LDL cholesterol undergoes oxidative modification when attacked by free radicals. Many experts believe that this modification accelerates plaque buildup in the arteries. This may help to explain why cigarette smokers—who have much higher levels of free radicals than nonsmokers—are more prone to suffer heart attacks.

Many laboratory studies have shown that adding vitamin E to plasma helps LDL cholesterol to resist oxidation. Recent research suggests that this effect on vitamin E (and, perhaps, the other antioxidants) may help prevent coronary heart disease in humans. Of thousands of people studied worldwide, those who consumed more antioxidants, either dietary or supplementary, were less likely to develop heart disease. In the chapters on specific antioxidants, we look more closely at the results of this research.

CANCER

The other major disease linked to damage from free radicals is cancer. While we do not completely understand the mechanism involved, many scientists believe that high levels of free radicals may play a role in transforming healthy cells into cancer cells. Free radicals may be involved in the development of cancers related to cigarette smoking, radiation, and chemical and physical carcinogens (such as asbestos). Some experts think that these cancers result from oxidative damage to DNA within the cells, resulting in mutations that perpetuate the production of abnormal DNA. This may be the first step in what is known to be a long, multistage progression from initial mutation to malignant cell.

Antioxidants seem to help most in cancers linked to free radical damage—especially those involving the gastrointestinal tract (colon, stomach, esophagus, and oropharynx) and the lungs. Many studies show that antioxidants can block this kind of DNA damage. Even after damage has occurred, antioxidants may be able to reverse some of the changes, or at least halt the long progression from simple DNA damage to development of cancer (although it is unlikely that the process can be stopped or reversed by antioxidants once an actual cancer has developed).

CATARACTS

Antioxidants appear to play an important role in preventing cataracts. Proteins, called *crystallins*, give the lens of the eye its transparency, making it the only clear organ in the body. When damaged by chronic exposure to the sun's ultraviolet rays (a potent generator of free radicals), the crystallins clump. This makes the lens opaque and causes blurred vision. The opaque area is the cataract.

Many studies have shown that increased amounts of dietary or supplementary antioxidants can reduce the risk of developing cataracts. Since cataract operations are the most common surgical procedure performed in the United States, this finding could have important economic implications. It could also provide tremendous relief from personal stress and inconvenience.

Some eye specialists believe that antioxidants may help prevent an even more serious eye disorder called macular degeneration, which causes severe visual impairment and can lead to permanent blindness. Years of free radical damage may be partly responsible for this condition, which affects up to 30 percent of the people in the United States ages 65 years and older. If free radicals are involved, antioxidants may play a protective role.

AGING AND DEPRESSED IMMUNE FUNCTION

In the mid-1950s, Dr. Denham Harman suggested that free radical reactions throughout life could cause the cumulative damage and deficits often associated with aging. Now that we have the technological ability to measure free radical damage and the effects of antioxidants on free radicals, more physicians are beginning to accept the possibility that Dr. Harman's theory may be correct. Unfortunately, the government's RDAs are not always sensitive to aging concerns. Some guidelines, for instance, give one RDA for people up to the age of 50 and another for those 51 and older. Clearly, dividing people into just two groups is a vast oversimplification. A person who is 51 years old has very different nutritional needs than someone who is 91.

Many laboratory experiments have linked free radicals to the age-related decline in immune function. Free radicals stimulate the body to produce and release larger amounts of *prostaglandins*, substances that can hamper some immune responses, particularly to infection. Studies show that vitamin E can reduce levels of prostaglandins. Some scientists believe that vitamin E accomplishes this by "neutralizing" free radicals.

Immune function usually appears to decline with age, but antioxidants may slow the rate of decline or even reverse it. In fact, many of the conditions we associate with aging may not be entirely related to aging.

The Future

With improving technology and expanding scientific information, researchers are looking to see if free radicals are causing or influencing a wider array of chronic diseases, and if antioxidants could prevent or ameliorate them. Among the diseases being studied are diabetes, Parkinson's disease, and Lou Gehrig's disease. Other studies, on free radicals in relation to exercise-related muscle injuries and the impact of antioxidants on recovery, may bring insights that will help maintain muscle function not only for athletes, but for the aging population.

As we improve our understanding of the role of free radicals in developing chronic diseases, and as we increase our knowledge of how micronutrients like vitamins E and C and beta-carotene can contribute to health, we can provide more specific, targeted recommendations for dietary intakes. We will show you how to put this information to work in upcoming chapters.

VITAMIN A

Vitamin A is not just a single nutrient, but a group of compounds that are structurally related and act in similar biological ways. The group includes two general categories: retinoids (preformed vitamin A) and carotenoids (precursors of vitamin A).

Whether you consume vitamin A in its preformed state or your body manufactures it from precursors, your liver stores it and your body uses it as needed. Because of this, you do not necessarily need to consume vitamin A every day. Also because of this, excessive amounts of vitamin A can accumulate in your body and lead to troublesome—even dangerous—toxic side effects.

The carotenoids got their name in the 1930s, when they were first discovered in carrots. Since then, more than 500 carotenoids have

Forms of Vitamin A

The body can use *retinoids*, vitamin A in its preformed state, immediately upon consumption. For that reason, retinoids—also called *retinol, retinaldehyde,* or *retinoic acid*—are considered "active" forms of vitamin A. Retinoids are fat-soluble: they dissolve in liquid fats but not in water. They are found naturally only in foods of animal origin, not in plants.

Carotenoids were once thought to be only the building blocks for vitamin A. But as you'll read later in this chapter, research has shown that they have important nutritional properties of their own. These substances have received increasing attention in recent years.

been identified. Carotenoids, the pigments that give plant life its red, orange, and yellow hues, are plentiful in many common fruits and vegetables, from sweet potatoes to apricots, from cantaloupes to carrots. Large amounts of beta-carotene—the best-known carotenoid, and the most abundant and most important nutritionally—are found in yellow and orange fruits and vegetables in particular. In contrast to retinoids, carotenoids exist only in plants.

Your body can change about 50 of the carotenoids identified so far into vitamin A. This conversion must take place before the carotenoids can be used or stored in the liver. Enzymes in the intestines divide the beta-carotene molecule, for example, into molecules of vitamin A, allowing the body to use the beta-carotene soon after it enters the bloodstream.

To meet your body's vitamin A requirements, you can consume either preformed retinoids or carotenoids such as beta-carotene.

History

Scientists have known of the existence of "vitamin A" for centuries (although only recently by that name). More than 3,500 years ago, writers described a connection between night blindness and a deficiency in foods that we now know are rich in vitamin A. Egyptian documents traced back to 1500 BC discuss treating night blindness with the juice squeezed from roasted or fried animal livers, foods that are particularly rich in vitamin A. These ancient references advise applying the juice directly upon the eyes themselves. During the 3rd and 4th centuries BC, Hippocrates suggested the better method of eating beef liver as a treatment for night blindness.

Early in the 20th century, researchers working with animals determined that specific nutritional substances were necessary for growth and survival. These studies showed that at least one of the substances—later identified as vitamin A—could be found in foods such as egg yolks and cod liver oil. A Swiss scientist first described the precise structure of vitamin A itself in 1930.

Like vitamin A itself, beta-carotene is fat-soluble. It has some distinct advantages over vitamin A, however, especially with respect to toxicity. For one thing, beta-carotene itself is nontoxic. For another, the body can decrease conversion of beta-carotene to vitamin A when blood levels of vitamin A are high. When you increase your intake of vitamin A and beta-carotene, the body's conversion process automatically slows down.

Basic Functions

• Vitamin A is essential for proper functioning of the light-sensitive portion of the eye, the retina (thus the name *retinoids*). This vitamin helps to form the pigments that make vision possible. Each time your eyes are exposed to light, you use the vitamin A-rich compounds in these pigments. Without enough vitamin A, vision in dim light worsens and you experience night blindness.

• Vitamin A is essential to the growth and maintenance of the tissues lining the body's surfaces—the skin, the trachea, the lungs, and the digestive, reproductive, and urinary tracts, for example. Vitamin A deficiency can lead to problems in these lining tissues, also known as epithelial tissues. The tissues will stop producing mucus (the substance that helps preserve and lubricate the body) and instead begin secreting a hard protein called keratin. This dries out and toughens the epithelial tissues and makes the body—including the eyes, throat, lungs, and digestive tract—more vulnerable to infections.

• Vitamin A appears to be necessary for normal bone growth and development, although its role in this process is not well understood.

• Vitamin A can make your immune system more responsive, so your body can better resist infection and, perhaps, such diseases as cancer. Studies show that vitamin A therapy can reduce deaths from measles and respiratory illnesses, for example. This protective effect is probably at least partly based on vitamin A's role in maintaining the health of your skin and other natural barriers that can keep out infection. Debate still exists, however, about the precise nature of vitamin A's role in this process.

• A growing number of studies now show that high levels of vitamin A and/or beta-carotene in the diet reduce the risk of cancer. This seems to be related to several properties of vitamin A and/or beta-carotene: the capacity to boost the immune system, the ability to keep epithelial tissues healthy (thus interfering with the process by which many cancers develop), and beta-carotene's function as an antioxidant.

• In both men and women, vitamin A promotes the normal workings of the reproductive system. It assists in pregnancy and lactation, although the reasons for this are still unclear.

Signs of Deficiency

Because the liver can store vitamin A, signs and symptoms may not appear with occasional dietary deficiencies. Problems have been observed with chronic deficiencies, however.

In the condition called *follicular hyperkeratosis*, one result of a vitamin A deficiency, the body's epithelial tissues produce too much of the hard protein keratin. When this happens on the skin, goose bump-like deposits of keratin form around hair follicles—typically on the shoulders, neck, back, buttocks, arms, and legs. Eventually, as the condition worsens, the skin assumes a rough, "toad-skin" texture. Excessive keratin production may also involve the epithelial cells of vital internal organs. In the respiratory tract, mucous secretions essential for carrying foreign bodies out of the lungs may decline. If the nose and mouth are affected, the senses of smell and taste can be lost. Weight loss and loss of appetite also appear to be related to keratinization of the tongue.

Night blindness is an early and reversible symptom of vitamin A deficiency. A deficiency of vitamin A can also cause irreversible eye conditions, however. Eyes commonly dry out, often leading to ulcerations of the cornea.

Who's at Risk for Vitamin A Deficiency?

If you answer yes to any of the following questions, you (or your child) have an above-average risk of developing a vitamin A deficiency.

• *Do you have chronic diarrhea, chronic pancreatitis, cystic fibrosis, or chronic liver disease (including hepatitis, cirrhosis, or liver cancer)?* Chronic diarrhea reduces the absorption of vitamin A. Liver diseases can reduce the amount of vitamin A stored by the body.

• *Do you consume large amounts of alcohol?* This reduces the levels of vitamin A and/or beta-carotene in the liver.

• *Do you smoke cigarettes?* Cigarette smoking decreases the level of beta-carotene in the blood.

• *Do you regularly take any medications that can interfere with your body's absorption of vitamin A from the intestinal tract?* These include certain drugs within the following categories: (1) cholesterol-lowering medications (colestipol and cholestyramine); (2) mineral oil (which attaches itself to vitamin A and carries it out through the intestinal tract); and (3) birth-control pills (which increase levels of retinol in the bloodstream and decrease liver stores of the vitamin which may increase the body's vitamin A needs).

• *Are you under a lot of stress?* Stress can reduce the level of retinol in the blood, probably by increasing the number of free radicals present and possibly by causing the body to break down vitamin A more quickly. Stress caused by overwork, fatigue, a fever, a chronic infection, or even too much exercise can have this effect on vitamin A levels.

• *Are you pregnant or breast-feeding?* If so, your body needs more vitamin A than usual.

• *Does your child avoid foods that are good sources of vitamin A?* Because of their rapid growth and faster metabolism, youngsters probably require more vitamin A, on a pound-for-pound basis, than adults do.

Vitamin A deficiency in children can retard growth, although the reasons for this are unclear. Scientists do know that the vitamin helps bones to develop normally, and when it is deficient, the bones stop growing. Rapid weight loss can also occur.

Deficiency-related problems of reproduction may involve deteriorated functioning of the testes, impaired sperm, spontaneous abortion, abnormal menses, or malformed offspring.

Because vitamin A plays a role in immunity, deficiencies can increase vulnerability to certain types of infections, particularly in the respiratory tract. Sore throats, sinus infections, and ear infections can also occur.

Vitamin A deficiency can result in poor enamel formation, making the teeth more vulnerable to decay.

Toxicity

If you consume more vitamin A than your body needs, your liver will store the excess, providing a ready reserve for days when you take too little vitamin A. Too much vitamin A accumulated in your body, unfortunately, can cause toxic side effects, a condition called hypervitaminosis A.

Your liver generally stores about 90 percent of the vitamin A in your body. When it reaches its capacity, however, vitamin levels in your blood begin to creep up. Large amounts of this nutrient in both the liver and the blood can contribute to toxic symptoms.

When toxicity does occur, it is usually the result of too many vitamin A supplements. Few foods contain enough preformed vitamin A to cause problems on their own. One of the best-known exceptions is liver—particularly polar bear liver, which contains 13,000 to 18,000 IU per gram and has been associated with toxicity problems when consumed by humans—but few people eat enough liver to cause trouble.

Older adults appear to have increased toxic risks, due to reasons such as decreased clearance of Vitamin A from their blood, compared to young or middle-aged adults. Even so, infants and children tend to be far more susceptible than adults to vitamin A overdose problems; youngsters typically experience difficulties at much lower doses, and symptoms are likely to be more pronounced. The signs of toxicity can also differ between adults and children. (See "Vitamin A Toxicity: Signs and Symptoms.") Preg-

Vitamin A Toxicity: Signs and Symptoms

Acute

Children	Adults
bulging fontanelle (soft spot on an infant's skull)	blurred vision
	drowsiness
	headaches
irritability	irritability
lethargy	loss of appetite
loss of appetite	muscular weakness
	skin scaling and peeling
	vomiting

Chronic

Children	Adults
bone pain	blurred vision
bulging fontanelle	bone pain
loss of appetite	diarrhea
premature bone closure	edema
stunted growth	enlargement of the liver and spleen
	fissures of the lips
	hair loss
	irritability
	itching
	lethargy
	loss of appetite
	menstrual irregularity
	skin scaling and peeling
	weight loss

nant women should take vitamin A only under the supervision of a doctor, since large doses have been associated with spontaneous abortions and birth defects (malformation of the head, face, heart, and nervous system).

The only side effect of high beta-carotene consumption is not dangerous: if you eat too many carrots (or other foods high in beta-carotene), you may develop a yellowish orange discoloration of the skin called *hypercarotenodermia*. This condition disappears within weeks once you cut your dosage of beta-carotene, and should not have any permanent adverse effects.

Health Merits

The body of evidence supporting health benefits for vitamin A and its precursor, beta-carotene, is growing rapidly. Many benefits have to do with the role of vitamin A (regardless of source) in the body's biochemical and physiological processes at a cellular level. Others have to do with the antioxidant powers of beta-carotene.

CANCER

Studies show that beta-carotene may protect against certain types of cancer, particularly cancers of the cervix, stomach, esophagus, and throat. Other studies suggest that beta-carotene may protect against cancers of the breast, ovary, colon, and prostate, although this evidence is currently less persuasive.

LUNG CANCER

• In one of the earliest and most persuasive studies—a 19-year evaluation of 1,954 middle-aged employees of the Western Electric Company in Chicago—researchers found that individuals who consumed the least amount of carotenes were seven times more likely to contract lung cancer than those who consumed the most. Of the 33 men who developed lung cancer during this study, 25 were in the lower half of carotene intake. The same study found that preformed vitamin A itself did not decrease the chances of developing lung cancer; the benefits came solely from carotenes.

• Johns Hopkins researchers, in a study that began in 1974 and was published in 1991, obtained and froze blood samples of 25,000 residents of Washington County, Maryland. Over the ensuing 15 years, the researchers measured the amounts of antioxidants in the blood samples, comparing levels in the 99 people who had developed lung cancer to levels in individuals who remained cancer-free. On average, the amounts of beta-carotene in the blood specimens of individuals with cancer were 16 percent lower than in those without cancer. Those who had the lowest levels of beta-carotene in their blood were 2.2 times more likely to develop lung cancer than those with the highest levels.

• One other study concerning vitamin A and cancer is important. In 1994, researchers at the U. S. National Cancer Institute and the National Public Health Institute in Finland reported on a lengthy study of 29,133 Finnish men. In that study, long-term smokers were divided into four groups: one group took only beta-carotene (20 mg per day); another, only vitamin E (50 mg per day); a third, both vitamins; and a fourth, a placebo.

Some of the study's conclusions were surprising—particularly the finding that beta-carotene and vitamin E do not offer smokers any protection from lung cancer. Even more startling was the suggestion that beta-carotene increases the risk of lung cancer among cigarette users by 18 percent. Other findings suggested a rise in the risk of stroke and heart disease in the beta-carotene group.

The study's authors and other authorities could not explain their findings, particularly those surrounding the increased risks associated with beta-carotene, which had always been considered safe. An editorial accompanying the study pointed out that the conclusions about lung cancer "may simply have been due to an extreme play of chance, since the finding is so much at variance with the totality of other evidence suggesting a benefit." Certainly that is a possibility.

We do not think that any study—no matter how large or how carefully conducted—can or should undermine all of the research that has preceded it. Much of this earlier research has been highly persuasive regarding the positive effects of beta-carotene. Of some 200 published reports on beta-carotene, most have shown benefits. One new study alone cannot refute that large body of evidence.

STOMACH CANCER

• A Swiss study, published in 1991, followed 2,974 men for 12 years, beginning in the early 1970s. Researchers found that men with low levels of carotenoids more frequently died from cancer. This was particularly true of stomach cancer; carotene levels were nearly 60 percent higher in survivors than in individuals who died of stomach cancer.

CERVICAL CANCER

• Researchers at the Fred Hutchinson Cancer Research Center and the University of Washington, Seattle, analyzed the diets of 189 women diagnosed with cancer of the cervix and compared them to a control group of 227 cancer-free women. In 1989, the researchers reported that high intakes of beta-carotene were associated with a reduced chance of developing this cancer. The intake of preformed vitamin A showed no protective effect against cervical cancer.

BREAST CANCER

• A British study drew and froze blood from 5,004 women and then followed them for several years; 39 developed breast cancer during that time. In 1984, researchers from St. Bartholomew's Hospital, London, evaluated the original blood samples and reported that beta-carotene levels in the blood of women without cancer were nearly 50 percent higher than levels in women with breast cancer.

PRECANCEROUS ORAL LESIONS

• In 1991, researchers at the University of Arizona studied the effect of high doses of beta-carotene on leukoplakia (whitish precancerous lesions) of the mouth. They treated 24 patients with 30 mg of beta-carotene per day for three to six months each. Leuko-plakia lesions regressed partially or completely in 71 percent of these patients.

CARDIOVASCULAR DISEASE

• Since 1980, Harvard researchers have been following 87,245 female nurses. In 1991, they reported that high intakes of caro-tenes were associated with a decreased risk of heart attack. The women who consumed the most beta-carotene had 22 percent fewer heart attacks than those who consumed the least.

• In a study that began in 1982, Harvard researchers have been following nearly 40,000 male physicians (ages 40 to 75). According to data published in 1990, of the 333 men identified as having heart disease at the beginning of the study (having previously undergone angioplasty or coronary bypass surgery), those taking a 50 mg supplement of beta-carotene every other day had 44 per-cent less risk of having a major cardiovascular event (such as a heart attack or stroke) than those who received a placebo.

• In another study in the Boston area published in 1992, research-ers followed nearly 1,300 older men and women for close to five years. Those who consumed the most beta-carotene were found to have 75 percent less risk of suffering a fatal heart attack than those who consumed the least.

IMMUNE DISORDERS

Some of the most interesting research into vitamin A and beta-carotene involves patients whose immune systems are not func-tioning properly, particularly people with AIDS (acquired immune deficiency syndrome).

AIDS

• John Hopkins researchers compared vitamin A levels in 126 individuals who tested positive for HIV (human immunodeficien-cy virus, which causes AIDS) and 53 who tested negative; all were considered at risk for HIV infection. The study, published in 1993, revealed that those people who tested negative for infection with the virus had vitamin A levels in their blood that were about 25 percent higher than those who tested positive. Among the HIV-positive group, deaths in subsequent years were six times greater in vitamin A-deficient individuals than in individuals with adequate intakes of the vitamin.

EYE DISORDERS

Researchers are finding that beta-carotene has a protective effect against common eye disorders such as cataracts and macular degeneration.

CATARACTS

• A 1991 study at Tufts University and other Boston-area institutions looked at carotene levels in the blood of both cataract patients (77 men and women) and cataract-free individuals (35 men and women). The risk for cataracts was significantly higher in those people with low beta-carotene levels. Individuals in the lowest 20 percent of beta-carotene measurements had five times more chance of developing cataracts than those in the top 20 percent.

• Researchers in Finland examined 47 men and women with cataracts and 94 without this eye disorder. All the subjects were ages 40 to 83 years old. According to data published in 1992, researchers at the University of Tampere found that both men and women in the lowest third of blood levels of beta-carotene had a 70 percent higher risk of developing cataracts than those in the highest two-thirds.

MACULAR DEGENERATION

• Macular degeneration—damage or breakdown of the macula (a part of the retina)—is the leading cause of blindness in people 65 years and older. Researchers have examined the theory that oxidative damage to the macula (the part of the retina that produces fine images) gradually causes it to break down. Because of beta-carotene's antioxidant activity, a 1993 study was conducted involving more than 1,000 individuals. Those with the highest levels of carotenoids in their blood were only one-third as likely to develop macular degeneration as those with the lowest levels.

How Much Vitamin A Do You Need?

The Recommended Dietary Allowance (RDA) for vitamin A varies, depending on age and sex. Current RDAs for vitamin A are expressed in retinol equivalents (RE), the measurement formally used in RDA tables, as well as in International Units (IU). Vitamin manufacturers most often use IUs on their labels.

Recommended Dietary Allowances

	RE (*in mcg*)*	IU
Infants		
0–12 months	375	1,875
Children		
1–3 years	400	2,000
4–6 years	500	2,500
7–10 years	700	3,500
Male Adolescents and Adults		
11+ years	1,000	5,000
Female Adolescents and Adults		
11+ years	800	4,000
Pregnant Women		
	800	4,000
Lactating Women		
first 6 months	1,300	6,500
second 6 months	1,200	6,000

* *Mcg stands for micrograms of retinol (or vitamin A), sometimes abbreviated as RE (retinol equivalents). 1 RE (1 mcg of retinol) equals 6 mcg of beta-carotene.*

Optimal Daily Allowance of Vitamin A and Beta-Carotene

We designed our strategy for vitamin A intake to provide you with the maximum benefits of this important nutrient, while minimizing the risk of toxic side effects. The first and most important step is to keep your intake of preformed vitamin A well below the level that would produce adverse effects. With safety in mind, we recommend an optimal dose of 1,000 mcg of RE, or 5,000 IU, of vitamin A per day.

Food Sources

Many common foods are rich in vitamin A. This important nutrient occurs naturally only in foods of animal origin, such as dairy products (milk, cheese, butter, and ice cream), egg yolks, fish (and fish oils), and liver and other internal organs. Other food products have been fortified with vitamin A, including margarine, breakfast cereals, and milk.

We obtain much of our vitamin A indirectly from the carotenoids, including beta-carotene, found in many vegetables and fruits—for instance, yellow and orange vegetables (carrots, sweet potatoes, and pumpkins), green leafy vegetables (spinach, broccoli, collard greens, turnip greens, and peppers), and yellow and orange fruits (papayas, oranges, apricots, peaches, and cantaloupes).

While nutrient tables are useful guides for vitamin A and beta-carotene intake, they are not always helpful for precise assessments. The amount of vitamin A in a product can vary, particularly in meat and dairy products, depending on the diet of the animal that the product came from. The content of carotenoids can vary, too, depending on growing conditions for the fruits and vegetables. The processing and storage of foods can also alter these values: both vitamin A and beta-carotene are insoluble in water; they are relatively unstable in heat; and exposure to light can destroy both of these nutrients.

But total quantity is only part of our recommendation. To avoid toxicity altogether, we believe everyone should obtain supplemental vitamin A through beta-carotene. When you rely on beta-carotene, you sidestep toxic risks and at the same time get the benefits of beta-carotene that are independent of vitamin A.

We recommend that you take 6 to 30 mg of beta-carotene per day. The results of studies vary as to how much beta-carotene might be optimal; for now, a dose of 15 mg seems to be a good compromise. You may want to move toward the higher end of the scale if you have a poor diet or have other risk factors for deficiency, however. In some people, particularly smaller ones, 20 to 30 mg of beta-carotene may produce yellowing of the skin; petite women may do best with a 15 mg dose. Note that 15 mg is equivalent to about 25,000 IU of vitamin A—much more than we recommend of the preformed nutrient itself.

Finally, if you take a supplement of beta-carotene to bring you up to our Optimal Daily Allowance (ODA), you do not need any supplemental vitamin A. You could take both—15 mg of beta-carotene and 1,000 mcg of RE, for example—but the beta-carotene alone will give you the optimal dose you need.

Vitamin A Content of Common Foods

Food Item	Amount of Vitamin A (in mcg of RE)
Acorn squash (½ cup, baked)	44
American cheese (1 oz)	82
Apricots (3 med, raw)	277
Asparagus (6 spears, boiled)	75
Avocado, California (½, med)	53
Avocado, Florida (½, med)	93
Beef liver (3½ oz, braised)	10,602
Beef soup, chunky (1 cup)	261
Beet greens (½ cup, boiled)	367
Blue cheese (1 oz)	65
Broccoli (½ cup, boiled)	110

Brussels sprouts (2, broiled) 56
Butter (1 tbsp) 114
Butternut squash (½ cup, boiled) 714
Camembert cheese (1 oz) 71
Cantaloupe (1 cup pieces) 516
Carrot (1 med) 2,025
Carrot juice (6 oz, canned) 4,738
Cheddar cheese (1 oz) 86
Chicken, breast (½, roasted) 26
Chicken, dark and light meat (3½ oz, roasted) 47
Chicken, leg (1, roasted) 45
Chicken liver (3½ oz, simmered) 4,913
Chicken soup, chunky (1 cup) 130
Chicken, thigh (1, roasted) 30
Clams (4 lg or 9 sm) 255
Colby cheese (1 oz) 78
Cottage cheese, low-fat (1 cup) 25
Cream of Wheat, instant (1 pkt) 375
Cream cheese (1 oz) 124
Egg (1 lg, boiled) 78
Figs (10, dried) 25
Gouda cheese (1 oz) 49
Grapefruit (½ med) 32
Green beans (½ cup, boiled) 41
Guava (1 med) 71
Haddock (3 oz, raw) 47
Halibut (3 oz, raw) 132
Herring (3 oz, raw) 80
Hubbard squash (½ cup, baked) 616
Ice milk, vanilla (1 cup) 52
Ice cream, vanilla (1 cup) 133
Kale (½ cup, boiled) 481
Lobster (3 oz, cooked) 74
Mackerel (3 oz, raw) 140
Mango (1 med) 806
Manhattan clam chowder (1 cup) 329

Marinara sauce (1 cup) 240
Milk, low-fat, 1% (8 oz)...145
Mozzarella cheese (1 oz)..68
Muenster cheese (1 oz)..90
Mustard greens (½ cup, boiled)..212
Nectarine (1 med) 100
Oatmeal, instant (1 pkt) 455
Okra (½ cup, boiled)..46
Orange (1 med) 26
Parsley (½ cup, raw) 156
Peach (1 med) 47
Peas (½ cup, boiled)..48
Provolone cheese (1 oz) 75
Prunes (10, dried) 167
Ricotta cheese, part skim (½ cup) 140
Sardines (2, canned in oil) 54
Sweet potato (1 med, baked) 2,488
Swiss chard (½ cup, boiled)..276
Swiss cheese (1 oz)...72
Swordfish (3 oz, raw) 101
Tangerine (1 med)...77
Tomato (1 med) 139
Tomato juice (6 oz)..101
Trout (3 oz, raw)..49
Turnip greens (½ cup, boiled) 213
Vegetarian soup, chunky (1 cup)..588
Yogurt, low-fat (8 oz) 36

BETA-CAROTENE CONTENT OF COMMON FOODS

Food Item	*Amount of Nutrient (in mg)*
Apricot, canned, drained (½ cup)	1.70
Apricot, dried (7 halves)	4.31
Apricot, raw (4)	17.62
Asparagus, raw (1 cup)	0.60
Beet greens (1 cup)	0.98

Broccoli, cooked (½ cup) 1.01
Cabbage, chinese, wild (1 cup) 0.37
Cantaloupe, raw (1 cup) 4.80
Carrot, cooked, canned, frozen (½ cup) 7.15
Carrot, raw (1 cup) 10.82
Cassava leaf (100 g) 3.00
Celery (1 cup) 0.85
Chicory leaf, raw (1 cup) 6.17
Coriander, not dried (1 cup)..0.32
Cress, leaf, raw (1 cup)... 2.08
Dill, not dried (1 cup)...0.40
Endive (1 cup) 0.65
Fennel leaves (1 cup) 4.01
Grapefruit, pink raw (½ med) 1.57
Green beans (1 cup)...0.69
Greens, collard (1 cup) 10.04
Greens, mustard (1 cup) 1.51
Guava, raw (¾ cup) 1.00
Kale (1 cup) 3.20
Leek, raw (1 cup) 1.04
Lettuce, iceberg (1 cup) 0.26
Lettuce, leaf (1 cup) 0.67
Lettuce, romaine (1 cup) 1.06
Mango, raw (½) 1.33
Mint, not dried (5 g) 0.37
Mushroom, chanterelle, raw (100 g) 1.30
Parsley, not dried (5 sprigs) 0.26
Peach, dried (1) 2.31
Pepper, red (1 cup) 3.30
Plum, raw (2) 0.55
Pumpkin (¾ cup) 2.70
Roquette, raw (100 g) 3.46
Rose hip puree, canned (100 g)..0.42
Scallion, raw (1 cup)..0.85
Spinach, cooked, drained (½ cup) 4.95
Spinach, raw (1 cup).. 2.30

Squash, summer (1 cup) 0.55

Squash, winter, cooked (¾ cup) 3.69

Squash, winter, raw (¾ cup)..0.71

Sweet potato, cooked (⅓ cup) 3.99

Swiss chard, raw (1 cup) 1.31

Tomato catsup (1 tbsp)..0.85

Tomato juice, canned (1 cup)... 2.20

Tomato sauce, canned (½ cup) 1.23

Tomato, raw (1 cup) 0.94

Tomato paste, canned (2 oz) 0.96

How Much Vitamin A Are People in the United States Getting?

According to government statistics, people in the United States have recently increased their intake of vitamin A and carotene. This is largely because people are now eating more deep yellow vegetables. Vitamin A fortification in food items such as margarine and dairy products is also partly responsible.

According to the most recent available statistics from the U.S. Department of Agriculture's Continuing Survey of Food Intakes by Individuals, for the years 1985 and 1986, women take an average 832 RE of vitamin A per day, which is close to the RDA. Consumption varies considerably from person to person, however. According to these data, the average woman consumes 1.5 mg of beta-carotene per day, far below the 6.0 mg per day necessary to meet U.S. Department of Agriculture and National Cancer Institute guidelines, and to meet our minimum ODA.

Other studies have also looked at whether people in the United States are meeting their needs for vitamin A. Data released in the 1980s showed that only 20 percent of the individuals surveyed for the Second National Health and Nutrition Examination Survey (NHANES II) ate any fruits or vegetables rich in beta-carotene on the day they were questioned.

How Much Vitamin A Are You Getting?

Before you decide that you need to take vitamin supplements or change the way you eat, you should know where you stand and how much improvement you really need. To help you analyze your current diet, we've developed a system you can use to calculate your approximate vitamin A and beta-carotene intake. (You'll find this same system in the other vitamin and mineral chapters, too.) Following are lists of food sources of vitamin A and beta-carotene, arranged according to the percentage of our Optimal Daily Allowance contained in them. The ODA for vitamin A is 1,000 mcg of RE; for beta-carotene, it is 6 to 30 mg. For this self-test, we have used an ODA of 15 mg of beta-carotene.

To determine your average daily intake of vitamin A and beta-carotene, start by keeping an accurate food diary for three or four days. The longer you keep the diary, the more accurate your calculations will be. Write down exactly what you eat and drink, together with an estimate of the serving size. Don't concern yourself with precisely how much vitamin A or beta-carotene each food item contains; simply use the charts to find the food item and the percentage of the ODA that it provides. Then add up all these percentages to see if you reach 100 percent each day.

If a particular item in your meals is missing from this chart (it would be impossible to include every food here), use the nutritional information on the food packaging. Many packaged foods list their vitamin A and beta-carotene contents right on the label.

After you've determined how much vitamin A and beta-carotene you are obtaining from your diet each day, you can calculate whether you need to take supplements to reach the ODA. If you've decided that your optimal dose of beta-carotene falls somewhere besides 15 mg in our recommended range (from 6 to 30 mg), take that into account when you calculate percentages. For example, 1 cup of canned tomato juice contains 10 percent of the beta-carotene you would need for an ODA of 15 mg. If your ODA is 30 mg, that same cup of tomato juice would fulfill only 5 percent of your needs.

After you've determined how much vitamin A and beta-carotene you are obtaining from your diet each day, you can calculate whether you need to take supplements to reach the ODA. Let's say that you determine that you are getting 50 percent of your vitamin A target through diet alone. You are consuming 500 mcg of vitamin A in your diet (50 percent x 1,000 mcg = 500 mcg). To make up the difference, we would advise you to supplement your diet with 500 mcg of vitamin A in tablet form (1,000 mcg – 500 mcg = 500 mcg).

Before finalizing your plan, review our advice in "Optimal Daily Allowance." Remember: if you take a beta-carotene tablet to raise your intake to your ODA for that nutrient, you don't need a supplemental vitamin A tablet. Yes, you can take both, but only beta-carotene is required.

PERCENTAGE OF VITAMIN A ODA
5 Percent

American cheese (1 oz)
Asparagus (6 spears, boiled)
Avocado, California (½ med)
Avocado, Florida (½ med)
Blue cheese (1 oz)
Brussels sprouts (4, boiled)
Camembert (1 oz)
Cheddar cheese (1 oz)
Colby cheese (1 oz)
Egg (1 lg, boiled)
Guava (1 med)
Herring (3 oz, raw)
Ice milk, vanilla (1 cup)
Lobster (3 oz, cooked)
Mozzarella cheese (1 oz)
Muenster cheese (1 oz)
Provolone cheese (1 oz)
Sardines, canned in oil (2)

Swiss cheese (1 oz)
Tangerine (1 med)

10 Percent

Broccoli (½ cup, boiled)
Butter (1 tbsp)
Chicken soup, chunky (1 cup)
Cream cheese (1 oz)
Halibut (3 oz, raw)
Ice cream, vanilla (1 cup)
Mackerel (3 oz, raw)
Milk, low-fat, 1% (8 oz)
Nectarine (1 med)
Parsley (½ cup, raw)
Prunes (10, dried)
Ricotta cheese, part skim (½ cup)
Swordfish (3 oz, raw)
Tomato (1 med)
Tomato juice (6 oz)

20 Percent

Apricots (3 med, raw)
Beef soup, chunky (1 cup)
Clams (4 lg or 9 sm)
Marinara sauce (1 cup)
Mustard greens (½ cup, boiled)
Swiss chard (½ cup, boiled)
Turnip greens (½ cup, boiled)

30 Percent

Beet greens (½ cup, boiled)
Bran Flakes cereal (1 oz)
Corn Flakes cereal (1 oz)
Cream of Wheat, instant (1 pkt)
Kale (½ cup, boiled)
Manhattan clam chowder (1 cup)
Oatmeal, instant (1 pkt)
Raisin Bran cereal (1 oz)

50 Percent

Cantaloupe (1 cup pieces)
Vegetable soup, chunky (1 cup)

60 Percent

Hubbard squash (½ cup, baked)

70 Percent

Butternut squash (½ cup, boiled)

80 Percent

Mango (1 med)

100 Percent or More

Beef liver (3½ oz, braised)
Breakfast cereals, most (1 oz)
Carrot (1 med)
Carrot juice, canned (6 oz)
Chicken liver (3½ oz, simmered)
Product 19 cereal (1 oz)
Sweet potato (1 med, baked)
Total cereal (1 oz)

PERCENTAGE OF BETA-CAROTENE ODA

5 Percent

Beet greens (1 cup)
Broccoli (½ cup, cooked)
Celery (1 cup)
Guava (¾ cup, raw)
Leek (1 cup, raw)
Lettuce, romaine (1 cup)
Mango (½, raw)
Mushroom, chanterelle (100 g, raw)
Scallion (1 cup, raw)
Swiss chard (1 cup, raw)
Tomato (1 cup, raw)

Tomato catsup (1 tbsp)
Tomato paste, canned (2 oz)
Tomato sauce, canned (½ cup)

10 Percent

Apricot, canned (½ cup, drained)
Cress leaf (1 cup, raw)
Grapefruit, pink (½ med, raw)
Greens, mustard (1 cup)
Peach (1, dried)
Pumpkin (¾ cup)
Spinach (1 cup, raw)
Tomato juice, canned (1 cup)

20 Percent

Apricot (7 halves, dried)
Cassava leaf (100 g)
Fennel leaves (1 cup)
Kale (1 cup)
Pepper, red (1 cup)
Roquette (100 g, raw)
Squash, winter (¾ cup, cooked)
Sweet potato (⅓ cup, cooked)

30 Percent

Cantaloupe (1 cup, cooked)
Spinach (½ cup, cooked, drained)

40 Percent

Carrot, canned, frozen (½ cup, cooked)
Chicory leaf (1 cup, raw)

60 Percent

Carrot (1 cup, raw)
Greens, collard (1 cup)

100 Percent or More

Apricot (4, raw)

Our Recommendations

HOW MUCH VITAMIN A AND BETA-CAROTENE DO YOU NEED TO ACHIEVE OPTIMAL HEALTH?

We advise that you consume 1,000 mcg of RE (5,000 IU) of vitamin A daily. For beta-carotene, we recommend 6 to 30 mg per day; for most people, 15 mg will meet optimal needs. Remember that taking a beta-carotene tablet to meet your ODA will also fulfill your vitamin A requirement; you do not need to take supplements of both.

WHAT SPECIAL CIRCUMSTANCES MIGHT AFFECT THE AMOUNT OF VITAMIN A AND BETA-CAROTENE YOU NEED TO TAKE?

You should be particularly conscientious about meeting the ODA for vitamin A if any of the following circumstances apply to you: you have one of certain chronic medical conditions (including diarrhea, liver disease, or pancreatitis); live a physically stressful life; are pregnant or breast-feeding; consume large amounts of alcohol; smoke cigarettes; or take particular medications (cholesterol-lowering drugs or birth-control pills). In addition, you should move toward the high end of our recommended ODA range (6 to 30 mg) for beta-carotene if you have any of these conditions.

IS IT POSSIBLE TO CONSUME THE OPTIMAL AMOUNT OF VITAMIN A AND BETA-CAROTENE THROUGH DIET ALONE?

It is possible to consume 1,000 mcg of vitamin A and 6 to 30 mg of beta-carotene each day solely through diet. Most people don't, however, and could benefit from supplementation.

VITAMIN B₃—NIACIN

Niacin was once a relatively obscure B vitamin, probably best known in medical circles as the vitamin that prevented pellagra, a disease with symptoms related to the skin, gastrointestinal system, and central nervous system. We now know that niacin is important for other reasons, too. In the 1980s, amid growing obsession with cholesterol, niacin emerged as a potentially powerful weapon in the battle against high blood cholesterol levels. Thousands of health-conscious people grabbed bottles of niacin tablets off the shelves of health food stores, convinced that they had finally found the magic pill to prevent diseased coronary arteries. That degree of optimism proved to be unjustified, but attention and respect for the vitamin grew as people saw niacin's potential role in helping to decrease blood cholesterol.

Forms of Niacin

The name niacin is commonly applied to two natural, active compounds: nicotinic acid and nicotinamide (also called niacinamide). If you feel uneasy about the similarity of those names to nicotine, the addictive substance in tobacco, you're not alone. In fact, these compounds are not chemically related to the dangerous sound-alike. Because researchers feared that the public might confuse them, however, the more generic term niacin was used to represent both nicotinic acid and nicotinamide. Niacin is now accepted as the name for vitamin B₃.

Basic Functions

• In concert with a variety of enzymes, niacin participates in a variety of metabolic processes. It helps convert energy derived from carbohydrates, fats, and protein into a form that the body can use.

History

Both niacin and pellagra, the disease with which it has been tied historically, have interesting backgrounds. Pellagra has been recognized since the 18th century, long before niacin itself was identified and linked to the disorder. Pellagra is a disease of niacin deficiency, generally occurring among poor populations and affecting most cells in the body. Its symptoms include diarrhea, dermatitis, a swollen mouth and tongue, delirium, and, in some cases, death.

Pellagra is relatively rare today, but it afflicted about 200,000 Americans per year early in the 20th century. At that time, many scientists were convinced that an infectious agent was responsible for the disease. But they were wrong, and their attempts to identify a disease-causing microbe failed.

Ultimately, a government investigator, Joseph Goldberger, began to explore the possibility that a nutritional deficiency was to blame. He set up a study in Jackson, Mississippi, at an orphanage where pellagra was common. Goldberger found that he could wipe out this disease by feeding the children high-protein foods like meat, beans, and eggs. At first, he and others concluded that a protein deficiency caused pellagra. Eventually, however, they discovered niacin, the nutrient in those foods responsible for their positive effects.

Ironically, some of the high-protein foods used by Goldberger—particularly milk—contained little niacin. Those foods were rich in tryptophan, an amino acid that was converted to niacin in the body. We now know that the body's ability to convert tryptophan to niacin helps us meet our requirement for vitamin B₃.

• In large doses, niacin (specifically, nicotinic acid) positively affects fats in the blood: it can decrease total cholesterol, while increasing the HDL ("good") component of cholesterol.

Signs of Deficiency

A niacin deficiency, caused by low intake of both niacin and tryptophan, most prominently affects the skin, which becomes cracked, darkly pigmented, and scaly, particularly in areas exposed to sunlight (such as the backs of the hands, the forehead, and the neck).

This deficiency also causes diarrhea and affects the nervous system, often leading to irritability, anxiety, depression, tremors, muscle weakness, confusion, and disorientation. In the most severe cases, it can produce dementia and hallucinations.

Although pellagra is now rare, it still occurs in individuals with severe deficiencies, producing symptoms such as dermatitis, diarrhea, delirium, swelling of the mouth and tongue, and death.

Who's At Risk for Niacin Deficiency?

If you answer yes to any of the following questions, you have an above-average risk of developing a niacin deficiency.

• *Do you exercise?* The more energy you expend, the more niacin you need, because niacin plays a role in converting foods into energy.

• *Are you pregnant?* Because pregnant women require more energy, they need more niacin. The RDAs advise an additional 2 mg per day during pregnancy.

• *Are you breast-feeding?* Women who are nursing lose niacin in their breast milk and also expend more energy; thus they need extra niacin.

Individuals at risk for niacin deficiency generally live in parts of the world where both niacin- and tryptophan-rich foods are scarce and where diets are poor.

Toxicity

In general, the risk of niacin toxicity is low for doses contained in most vitamin supplements. Some people who use niacin to reduce blood cholesterol levels, however, have taken things to extremes— and paid the price. They've discovered that very high doses of niacin can produce uncomfortable—at times even dangerous— side effects. Other people have had the same trouble after self-prescribing excessive amounts of this vitamin to boost energy and stamina, a benefit unsubstantiated by scientific research.

The symptoms of high doses of niacin depend on the form of B$_3$ taken. Nicotinic acid can produce severe flushing, usually within an hour or two after consumption, because it stimulates the release of histamine, a substance that dilates the blood vessels. According to one study, 92 percent of people who take doses of 3 g per day experience this flushing. While this makes some individuals uncomfortable enough to discontinue use of the vitamin, many other people develop a tolerance or control the effect by taking aspirin or an antihistamine shortly before consuming a dose of nicotinic acid.

Other side effects associated with nicotinic acid include skin tingling, itching, stinging, rashes, headaches, dryness, nausea, and diarrhea. But physicians are particularly worried about more serious consequences of extremely high doses which can produce high blood sugar levels, ulcers, liver damage, or irregular heart rhythms.

A 3 g dose of nicotinic acid can double a person's risk of developing certain kinds of abnormal heart rhythms and is generally considered to be toxic. We strongly discourage levels that high without medical supervision; 3 g is a pharmacological dose, not a supplemental one. In other words, 3 g of niacin is no longer a vitamin, but a drug. Although you can purchase nicotinic acid in supermarkets and pharmacies without a prescription, you should take the potential risks of this substance seriously. Most doctors advise people with peptic ulcers to be particularly cautious in using nicotinic acid.

Fewer serious toxic risks have been associated with nicotinamide than with nicotinic acid, but problems can occur with either form of vitamin B_3. Heartburn, nausea, headaches, fatigue, sore throats, and dry hair have been reported in association with high doses of nicotinamide.

Health Merits

Niacin has been used to treat high blood cholesterol levels and pellagra.

CHOLESTEROL

Niacin can play a role in reducing blood cholesterol levels. This benefit usually requires very high doses, however. Acting like a drug (not a vitamin) when taken in high doses, nicotinic acid can reduce both total cholesterol and LDL ("bad") cholesterol. At the same time, it can increase HDL ("good") cholesterol and cut triglyceride levels. These changes significantly reduce the risk of coronary heart disease and heart attacks.

The evidence for this benefit is so persuasive that the Expert Panel of the National Cholesterol Education Program singled out nicotinic acid as one of two drugs that doctors should recommend first to control cholesterol levels. These experts were particularly impressed by studies that indicated a significant drop in the risk of heart disease corresponding to reduced cholesterol levels.

• One of the best-known clinical trials, dating back to the 1970s, was called the Coronary Drug Project. In this study, about 5,000 men with a history of coronary heart disease were randomly assigned to receive one of three treatments: (1) niacin, (2) a medication called clofibrate, or (3) a placebo. After five years, the group taking niacin (3 g per day) had the lowest average cholesterol levels—226 mg per dL. Those taking clofibrate had average measurements of 235, and those taking a placebo had 251. Another finding was just as impressive: the men taking niacin had fewer life-threatening episodes. Their percentage of coronary events (such as heart attacks) was 19.8 percent lower than in the placebo group, compared with a 9.5 percent reduction in the clofibrate group.

Again, however, we warn that decreasing cholesterol requires high doses of niacin—so high that you should take them only under a doctor's supervision. Your doctor will probably order periodic blood tests to be sure that the high doses are not adversely affecting your liver function. These visits to your doctor's office are extremely important and well worth the time and expense.

PELLAGRA

We've already discussed pellagra, a disease that can be prevented and treated with either nicotinic acid or nicotinamide. At the first signs of this deficiency disease, individuals usually receive up to 50 mg of vitamin B₃ as many as 10 times per day. The vitamin can also be given via injection.

SCHIZOPHRENIA

A few therapists have used nicotinamide to treat schizophrenia. A large body of scientific research has failed to substantiate niacin's value for this purpose, however.

How Much Niacin Do You Need?

The body's requirements for vitamin B₃ can be met in part by the conversion of tryptophan to niacin. Even so, most people need to consume additional niacin to meet the RDA guidelines.

Optimal Daily Allowance

To select an optimal daily allowance (ODA) of niacin, we examined the energy needs of men and women and chose a level to meet the needs of the most active individuals. We believe that 20 NE (niacin equivalent) per day—the highest RDA—is an optimal amount.

Recommended Dietary Allowances

	NE (in mg)

Infants

0–6 months 5

6–12 months 6

Children

1–3 years 9

4–6 years 12

7–10 years..13

Male Adolescents and Adults

11–14 years..17

15–18 years..20

19–50 years..19

51+ years 15

Female Adolescents and Adults

11–50 years..15

51+ years 13

Pregnant Women

....17

Lactating Women

....20

The quantitative measure officially used for niacin is niacin equivalents, NE per day—the highest RDA—is an optimal dose.

Niacin Content of Common Foods

Food Item	*Amount of Vitamin (in mg)*
Almonds (1 oz)	1.0
Anchovy (3 oz, raw)	11.9
Apricots (10 halves, dried)	1.0
Avocado, California (½ med)	1.6
Avocado, Florida (½ med)	2.9
Bacon (3 slices, fried)	1.4
Bagel (1)	1.9
Beef, bottom round (3½ oz, braised)	3.9
Beef, brisket (3½ oz, braised)	3.0
Beef soup, chunky (1 cup)	2.7
Beef, top round (3½ oz, broiled)	5.9
Broadbeans (1 cup, boiled)	1.2
Chicken, breast (½, roasted)	12.5
Chicken, dark and light meat (3½ oz, roasted)	8.5
Chicken, dark meat (3½ oz, roasted)	6.4
Chicken, leg (1, roasted)	7.1

Food Sources

Meats and nuts are good sources of niacin. So are poultry, fish, and whole-grain and enriched breads. Many cereals are also enriched with niacin.

Keep in mind that the amino acid tryptophan, after going through a conversion process in the body, also provides us with niacin. Milk, eggs, and corn have limited amounts of niacin in them but are good sources of tryptophan, and are therefore wise choices for maintaining a high niacin level.

Niacin is a stable vitamin and withstands high temperatures and exposure to oxygen. Because it dissolves in water, though, cooking in liquid will partially leach niacin content from food.

Chicken, light meat (3½ oz, roasted) 11.1
Chicken soup, chunky (1 cup) 4.4
Chicken, thigh (1, roasted) 3.9
Chicken, wing (1, roasted) 2.3
Clams (4 lg or 9 sm, raw)..1.5
Cod (3 oz, raw)..1.8
Corn (½ cup, boiled)...1.3
Corn tortilla (1)..1.5
Corned beef (3½ oz, cooked)..3.0
Crab (3 oz, cooked)...1.1
Cream of wheat, instant (1 pkt) 5.0
Figs (10, dried)..1.3
Flank steak (3½ oz, broiled)..4.8
Flounder (3½ oz, raw) 1.7
French bread (1 slice)...1.2
Great Northern beans (1 cup, boiled) 1.2
Ground beef, lean (3½ oz, baked)..4.3
Guava (1 med) 1.1
Halibut (3 oz, raw)...5.0
Ham (3½ oz, canned)...3.2
Herring (3 oz, raw) 2.7
Hot dog, beef (1) 1.4
Kidney beans (1 cup, boiled)..1.0
Lamb chop, loin (1, boiled)...3.1
Lamb chop, rib (1, broiled) 3.6
Leg of lamb (3 oz, roasted) 4.7
Lentils (1 cup, boiled)..2.1
Liver, beef (3½ oz, braised) 10.7
Liver, chicken (3½ oz, simmered)...4.5
Lobster (3 oz, cooked) 0.9
Lobster (3 oz, raw)...1.2
Mackerel (3 oz, raw)..7.4
Mango (1 med)...1.2
Manhattan clam chowder (1 cup) 1.8
Marinara sauce (1 cup)..4.0
Miso (½ cup)...1.2

Mushrooms (½ cup, raw)..1.4
Navy beans (1 cup, boiled)..1.0
Nectarine (1 med) 1.3
Oatmeal, instant (1 pkt) 5.5
Oysters (6 med, raw)..1.1
Peach (10 halves, dried)..5.7
Peanut butter (1 tbsp)..2.2
Peanuts (1 oz) 4.0
Pears (10 halves, dried)..2.4
Peas (½ cup, raw) 1.6
Pork, loin (3½ oz, roasted)..5.4
Pork, shoulder (3½ oz, roasted) 4.0
Potato (baked without skin)...2.2
Potato chips (1 oz)..1.2
Pretzels (1 oz) 1.2
Prune juice (8 oz, canned)..2.0
Prunes (10 dried)..1.6
Raisins, golden seedless (⅔ cup) 1.1
Rice, brown (1 cup, cooked) 2.7
Rice, white, enriched (1 cup, cooked) 2.1
Salmon (3 oz, raw)..6.7
Sardines (2, canned in oil) 1.3
Scallops (6 lg or 14 sm)...1.0
Shrimp (12 lg, raw) 2.2
Sole (3½ oz, raw) 1.7
Spaghetti, enriched (1 cup, cooked)......................................1.5
Sunflower seeds (1 oz, dried)...1.3
Swordfish (3 oz, raw) 8.2
Tomato juice (6 oz)..1.2
Tuna (3 oz, canned in water)..4.9
Turkey, dark and light meat (3½ oz, roasted) 5.1
Turkey, light meat (3½ oz, roasted) 6.3
Vegetable soup, chunky (1 cup)...1.2
White bread (1 slice)...0.9
Whole-wheat bread (1 slice)...1.0

How Much Niacin Are People in the United States Getting?

The government's Continuing Survey of Food Intakes by Individuals, with its most recent data collected in the mid-1980s, found that both men and women ages 19 to 50 consumed an average of 10.8 NE of niacin per day. Other studies have shown that the typical U.S. daily diet includes 700 mg of tryptophan for women (which provides 11.7 NE of niacin) and 1,100 mg for men (18.4 NE of niacin).

How Much Niacin Are You Getting?

Before you decide that you need to take vitamin supplements or change the way you eat, you should know where you stand and how much improvement you really need. To help you analyze your current diet, we've developed a system you can use to calculate your approximate niacin intake. (You'll find this system in the other vitamin and mineral chapters, too.) Following is a list of niacin food sources, arranged according to the percentage of our Optimal Daily Allowance (20 mg) of niacin contained in them. Since an 8 ounce glass of canned prune juice contains 2 mg of niacin and the ODA for niacin is 20 mg, we've listed prune juice in the 10 Percent category. (We have erred on the conservative side when rounding off percentages.)

To determine your average daily intake of niacin, start by keeping an accurate food diary for three or four days. The longer you keep the diary, the more accurate your calculations will be. Write down exactly what you eat and drink, together with an estimate of the serving size. Don't concern yourself with precisely how much niacin each food item contains; simply use the list to find the food item and the percentage of the ODA that it provides. Then add up all these percentages to see if you reach 100 percent each day.

If a particular item in your meals is missing from this chart (it would be impossible for us to include every food item here), use the nutritional information on the food packaging. Most packaged foods are required to list their vitamin contents on the label.

After you've determined how much niacin you are obtaining from your diet each day, you can calculate whether you need to take supplements to reach the ODA. Let's say that you determine that you are getting 50 percent of your niacin target through diet alone. You are consuming 10 mg of niacin in your diet (50 percent x 20 mg = 10 mg). To make up the difference, we would advise you to supplement your diet with 10 mg of niacin in tablet form (20 mg – 10 mg = 10 mg).

PERCENTAGE OF NIACIN ODA

5 Percent

Almonds (1 oz)
Apricots (10 halves, dried)
Avocado, California (½, med)
Bacon (3 slices, fried)
Bagel (1)
Broadbeans (1 cup, boiled)
Clams (4 lg or 9 sm, raw)
Cod (3 oz, raw)
Corn (½ cup, boiled)
Corn tortilla (1)
Crab (3 oz, cooked)
Dates (10, dried)
Figs (10, dried)
Flounder (3½ oz, raw)
French bread (1 slice)
Great Northern beans (1 cup, boiled)
Guava (1 med)
Hot dog, beef (1)
Kidney beans (1 cup, boiled)

Lobster (3 oz, cooked)
Mango (1 med)
Manhattan clam chowder (1 cup)
Miso (½ cup)
Mushrooms (½ cup, raw)
Navy beans (1 cup, boiled)
Nectarine (1 med)
Oysters (6 med, raw)
Peas (½ cup, boiled)
Potato chips (1 oz)
Pretzels (1 oz)
Prunes (10 dried)
Raisins, golden seedless (⅔ cup)
Sardines (2, canned in oil)
Scallops (6 lg or 14 sm)
Sole (3½ oz, raw)
Spaghetti, enriched (1 cup, cooked)
Sunflower seeds (1 oz, dried)
Tomato juice (6 oz)
Turkey breast (1 slice)
Vegetable soup, chunky (1 cup)
Wheat germ (¼ cup, toasted)
White bread (1 slice)
Whole-wheat bread (1 slice)

10 Percent

Avocado, Florida (½ med)
Beef, bottom round (3½ oz, braised)
Beef, brisket (3½ oz, braised)
Beef soup, chunky (1 cup)
Chicken, thigh (1, roasted)
Chicken, wing (1, roasted)
Corned beef (3½ oz, cooked)
Haddock (3 oz, raw)
Ham (3½ oz, canned)
Herring (3 oz, raw)
Lamb chop, loin (1, broiled)

Lentils (1 cup, boiled)
Peanut butter (1 tbsp)
Peanuts (1 oz)
Pear (10 halves, dried)
Potato (baked, with skin)
Potato (baked, without skin)
Prune juice (8 oz, canned)
Rice, brown (1 cup, cooked)
Rice, white, enriched (1 cup, cooked)
Shrimp (12 lg, raw)
Turkey, dark meat (3½ oz, roasted)

20 Percent

Beef, top round (3½ oz, broiled)
Bran Flakes cereal (1 oz)
Chicken soup, chunky (1 cup)
Corn Flakes cereal (1 oz)
Cream of Wheat, instant (1 pkt)
Flank steak (3½ oz, broiled)
Ground beef, lean (3½ oz, baked)
Halibut (3 oz, raw)
Leg of lamb (3 oz, roasted)
Liver, chicken (3½ oz, simmered)
Marinara sauce (1 cup)
Oatmeal, instant (1 pkt)
Peach (10 halves, dried)
Pork, shoulder (3½ oz, roasted)
Raisin Bran cereal (1 oz)
Tuna (3 oz, canned in water)
Turkey, light and dark meat (3½ oz, roasted)

30 Percent

Chicken, dark meat (3½ oz, roasted)
Chicken, leg (1, roasted)
Mackerel (3 oz, raw)
Salmon (3 oz, raw)
Turkey, light meat (3½ oz, roasted)

40 Percent

Chicken, light and dark meat (3½ oz, roasted)
Swordfish (3 oz, raw)

50 Percent

Anchovy (3 oz, raw)
Chicken, light meat (3½ oz, roasted)
Liver, beef (3½ oz, braised)

60 Percent

Chicken, breast (½, roasted)

100 Percent or More

Breakfast cereals, most (1 oz)
Product 19 cereal (1 oz)
Total cereal (1 oz)

Our Recommendations

HOW MUCH NIACIN DO YOU NEED TO ACHIEVE OPTIMAL HEALTH?

We advise consuming 20 mg of niacin per day, which is the highest of the RDAs.

WHAT SPECIAL CIRCUMSTANCES MIGHT AFFECT THE AMOUNT OF NIACIN YOU NEED TO TAKE?

If you exercise or if you are pregnant or breast-feeding, you should be particularly conscientious about consuming the optimal dose of niacin.

IS IT POSSIBLE TO CONSUME THE OPTIMAL AMOUNT OF NIACIN THROUGH DIET ALONE?

While you could consume 20 mg of niacin per day through diet alone, most people don't. The average person in the United States takes in only about half of our optimal recommendation. You may find it necessary to take a niacin supplement each day.

VITAMIN B$_6$—PYRIDOXINE

Scientists first firmly identified and described vitamin B$_6$ and its structure in 1939. Today we know that this vitamin exists naturally in foods in three closely related forms: pyridoxine, pyridoxal, and pyridoxamine. Nutrition supplements generally provide B$_6$ in the form of pyridoxine.

Basic Functions

• Vitamin B$_6$ is necessary to convert amino acids to proteins.

• Vitamin B$_6$ is important in forming tryptophan, an essential amino acid, and helps to convert tryptophan to niacin (vitamin B$_3$) in the body.

• Vitamin B$_6$ is important in forming hemoglobin, the oxygen-carrying component of red blood cells. It may also help red blood cells to function normally.

• Vitamin B$_6$ is involved in forming chemical messengers called neurotransmitters.

• Vitamin B$_6$ is necessary to convert sugars from the form in which the body stores them (as glycogen) to the form that the body can use for energy (glucose).

• Vitamin B$_6$ plays an as-yet unclear role in the utilization of fats.

Signs of Deficiency

Vitamin B$_6$ deficiencies are rare, thanks to the wide availability of this nutrient in everyday foods. When a deficiency does occur, the most frequent signs and symptoms include an impaired immune system, anemia, inflammation of the tongue and mucous membranes of the mouth, scaling skin, weakness, dizziness, nausea and vomiting, irritability, depression, and—especially in infants—convulsions.

Toxicity

Some case reports have shown that as few as 200 mg per day of vitamin B_6 can cause neurological problems, including numbness in the feet and hands and difficulty walking. Vitamin B_6 is safe for most people in doses of up to 500 mg per day (about 250 times the

---

Who's at Risk for Vitamin B_6 Deficiency?

If you answer yes to any of the following questions, you have an above-average risk of developing a vitamin B_6 deficiency.

• *Are you pregnant?* Women who are pregnant or have just given birth require extra vitamin B_6. The RDA suggests an additional 0.6 mg of B_6 during pregnancy.

• *Are you breast-feeding?* Women who breast-feed can lose as much as 0.25 mg of vitamin B_6 per liter of milk. The RDAs advise an additional 0.5 mg of B_6 per day when breast-feeding.

• *Are you taking certain drugs, such as isoniazid (to treat tuberculosis), hydralazine (for high blood pressure), or penicillamine (for rheumatoid arthritis)?* These drugs can increase the body's excretion of vitamin B_6 in the urine.

• *Are you taking birth-control pills?* Blood levels of vitamin B_6 decrease 15 to 20 percent in women taking birth-control pills. The reasons for this are not clear.

• *Does your diet include a lot of protein?* Vitamin B_6 plays an important role in protein metabolism, so the more protein you consume, the more vitamin B_6 you need.

• *Do you drink a lot of alcohol?* Some 20 to 30 percent of alcoholics experience a vitamin B_6 deficiency.

RDA for adult males), however. Toxic symptoms at doses above 500 mg include dermatitis (skin rash) related to sun exposure, difficulty walking, and numbness or tingling in the hands and feet. Symptoms tend to disappear when high doses are discontinued, although amounts of 2,000+ mg have been associated with permanent nerve damage.

Health Merits

If you've read the ads in health magazines, you may have seen claims that large doses of B_6 can alleviate depression, premenstrual syndrome (PMS), asthma, muscle fatigue, and even autism. But you shouldn't take these claims too seriously: scientific evidence does not support most of them. Proponents of B_6, for example,

Recommended Dietary Allowances

Infants

0–6 months	0.3 mg
6–12 months	0.6 mg

Children

1–3 years	1.0 mg
4–6 years	1.1 mg
7–10 years	1.4 mg

Male Adolescents and Adults

11–14 years	1.7 mg
15+ years	2.0 mg

Female Adolescents and Adults

11–14 years	1.4 mg
15–18 years	1.5 mg
19+ years	1.6 mg

Pregnant Women

	2.2 mg

Lactating Women

	2.1 mg

claim that doses of 50 to 200 mg can "cure" PMS. According to research studies, a placebo seems to be just as effective.

CORONARY HEART DISEASE

Vitamin B_6 may prove useful in helping to prevent coronary heart disease. According to a number of studies, B_6 decreases blood levels of an amino acid called homocysteine. This in turn decreases the risk of heart problems.

How Much Vitamin B_6 Do You Need?

The need for vitamin B_6 varies depending on factors described elsewhere in this book. Your requirements increase, for example, as your consumption of protein rises. The RDAs of B_6 have actually declined slightly in recent guideline revisions, but we still believe it is important to obtain optimal amounts. You can do this with little risk of toxic effects by following recommended intake levels.

Optimal Daily Allowance

We recommend 4 mg as the optimal daily allowance (ODA) of vitamin B_6. This is nearly double the highest-level RDA. We believe this higher level is appropriate for both men and women striving toward optimal health. This dose will help ensure reduced levels of the amino acid homocysteine, which may decrease the risk of heart problems. This dose will also compensate for any special circumstances discussed in the box, "Who's at Risk for Vitamin B_6 Deficiency?"

Vitamin B_6 Content of Common Foods

Food Item	Amount of Vitamin (in mg)
Acorn squash (½ cup, baked)	0.20
Anchovy (3 oz, raw)	0.12
Artichoke (1 med, boiled)	0.10

Asparagus (½ cup, boiled)...0.13
Avocado, California (½ med) 0.24
Avocado, Florida (½ med) 0.42
Banana (1 med) 0.66
Beef, bottom round (3½ oz, braised)...0.34
Beef, brisket (3½ oz, braised)..0.25
Beef soup, chunky (1 cup) 0.13
Beef, top round (3½ oz, broiled) 0.54
Black beans (1 cup, boiled) 0.12
Blackeye peas (1 cup, boiled)...0.17
Broadbeans (1 cup, boiled)..0.12
Broccoli (½ cup, boiled)..0.15
Brussels sprouts (4, broiled) 0.14
Butternut squash (½ cup, boiled) 0.13
Carp (3 oz, raw)..0.16
Carrot (1 med, raw) 0.11
Carrot juice (6 oz, canned)..0.40
Cauliflower (½ cup, boiled)..0.13
Chicken, breast (½, roasted) 0.57
Chicken, dark and light meat (3½ oz, roasted).........................0.40
Chicken, leg (1, roasted)...0.37
Chicken, thigh (1, roasted) 0.19
Chicken, wing (1, roasted)...0.14
Cod (3 oz, raw)...0.21

Food Sources

Many common foods are rich in vitamin B₆. If your diet includes liver, fish, pork, soybeans, wheat germ, peanuts, or walnuts, for example, you are getting B₆ in your meals. Dairy products, most vegetables, and fruits (with the exception of bananas) contain relatively little B₆.

When preparing foods, remember that vitamin B₆ is water-soluble, and significant amounts of vitamin B₆ can be lost in processing and cooking.

Cottage cheese, low-fat (1 cup)..0.15
Cream of wheat, instant (1 pkt) 0.50
Figs (10, dried)...0.42
Flank steak (3½ oz, broiled)..0.35
Garbanzo beans (1 cup, boiled) 0.23
Great Northern beans (1 cup, boiled) 0.21
Ground beef, lean (3½ oz, baked) 0.20
Haddock (3 oz, raw)..0.26
Halibut (3 oz, raw)..0.29
Ham (3½ oz, canned)...0.48
Hazelnuts (1 oz) 0.17
Herring (3 oz, raw) 0.26
Hubbard squash (½ cup, baked)..0.18
Kidney beans (1 cup, boiled)..0.21
Lentils (1 cup, boiled)...0.35
Lima beans (1 cup, boiled) 0.30
Liver, beef (3½ oz, braised)..0.91
Liver, chicken (3½ oz, simmered) 0.58
Mackerel (3 oz, raw)..0.34
Manhattan clam chowder (1 cup) 0.26
Milk, low-fat, 1% (8 oz)...0.11
Miso (½ cup) 0.30
Navy beans (1 cup, boiled)...0.30
Oatmeal, instant (1 pkt) 0.74
Onions (½ cup, raw) 0.13
Orange (1 med) 0.10
Peas (½ cup, boiled)..0.17
Pineapple juice (8 oz, canned)...0.24
Pinto beans (1 cup, boiled) 0.27
Pork, loin (3½ oz, roasted)...0.38
Pork, shoulder (3½ oz, roasted) 0.33
Potato (baked with skin)..0.70
Potato (baked without skin)...0.47
Potato chips (1 oz)...0.14
Prunes (10, dried)..0.22
Raisins, golden seedless (⅔ cup) 0.32

Salmon (3 oz, raw) 0.70
Sweet potato (1, baked)..0.28
Swordfish (3 oz, raw) 0.28
Tomato juice (6 oz)...0.20
Tuna (3 oz, canned in water)...0.32
Turkey, dark and light meat (3½ oz, roasted) 0.41
Vegetable soup, chunky (1 cup)...0.19
Wheat germ (¼ cup, toasted) 0.28

How Much Vitamin B₆ Are People in the United States Getting?

The average person in the United States consumes slightly less vitamin B₆ than the RDA. Government surveys in the mid-1980s found that men consumed an average of 1.87 mg of B₆ per day (0.13 short of the RDA), and women consumed an average of 1.16 mg (.44 short of the RDA).

How Much Vitamin B₆ Are You Getting?

Before you decide that you need to take vitamin supplements or change the way you eat, you should know where you stand and how much improvement you really need. To help you analyze your current diet, we've developed a system you can use to calculate your approximate vitamin B₆ intake. (You'll find this system in the other vitamin and mineral chapters, too.) Following is a list of vitamin B₆ food sources, arranged according to the percentage of our Optimal Daily Allowance (4 mg) of B₆ contained in them. (We have erred on the conservative side when rounding off percentages.)

To determine your average daily intake of vitamin B₆, start by keeping an accurate food diary for three or four days. The longer you keep the diary, the more accurate your calculations will be. Write down exactly what you eat and drink, together with an estimate of the serving size. Don't concern yourself with precisely how much vitamin B_6 each food item contains; simply use the chart to find the food item and the percentage of the ODA that it provides. Then add up all these percentages to see if you reach 100 percent each day.

If a particular item in your meals is missing from this list (it would be impossible for us to include every food item here), use the nutritional information on the food packaging. Most packaged foods are required to list their vitamin contents on the label.

After you've determined how much vitamin B_6 you are obtaining from your diet each day, you can calculate whether you need to take any supplements to reach the ODA. Let's say that you determine that you are getting 25 percent of your vitamin B_6 target through diet alone. You are consuming 1 mg of vitamin B_6 in your diet (25 percent x 4 mg = 1 mg). To make up the difference, we would advise you to supplement your diet with 3 mg of vitamin B_6 in tablet form (4 mg − 1 mg = 3 mg). Some multivitamin supplements will provide you with all the extra B_6 you need, so read labels carefully.

Percentage of Vitamin B_6 ODA

5 Percent

Acorn squash (½ cup, baked)
Avocado, California (½ med)
Beef, bottom round (3½ oz, braised)
Beef, brisket (3½ oz, braised)
Chicken, leg (1, roasted)
Cod (3 oz, raw)
Flank steak (3½ oz, broiled)
Garbanzo beans (1 cup, boiled)
Great Northern beans (1 cup, boiled)
Ground beef, lean (3½ oz, baked)
Haddock (3 oz, raw)
Halibut (3 oz, raw)
Herring (3 oz, raw)

Kidney beans (1 cup, boiled)
Lentils (1 cup, boiled)
Lima beans (1 cup, boiled)
Mackerel (3 oz, raw)
Manhattan clam chowder (1 cup)
Miso (½ cup)
Navy beans (1 cup, boiled)
Pineapple juice (8 oz, canned)
Pinto beans (1 cup, boiled)
Pork, loin (3½ oz, roasted)
Pork, shoulder (3½ oz, roasted)
Prunes (10, dried)
Raisins, golden seedless (⅔ cup)
Sweet potato (1, baked)
Swordfish (3 oz, raw)
Tuna (3 oz, canned in water)
Tomato juice (6 oz)
Wheat germ (¼ cup, toasted)

10 Percent

Avocado, Florida (1 med)
Banana (1 med)
Beef, top round (3½ oz, braised)
Bran Flakes cereal (1 oz)
Carrot juice (6 oz, canned)
Chicken, breast (½, roasted)
Chicken, dark and light meat (3½ oz, roasted)
Corn Flakes cereal (1 oz)
Cream of Wheat, instant (1 pkt)
Figs (10, dried)
Ham (3½ oz, canned)
Liver, chicken (3½ oz, simmered)
Oatmeal, instant (1 pkt)
Potato (baked with skin)
Raisin Bran cereal (1 oz)
Salmon (3 oz, raw)
Turkey, dark and light meat (3½ oz, roasted)

---

20 Percent

Liver, beef (3½ oz, braised)

---

50 Percent

Breakfast cereals, most (1 oz)
Product 19 cereal (1 oz)
Total cereal (1 oz)

Our Recommendations

HOW MUCH VITAMIN B_6 DO YOU NEED TO ACHIEVE OPTIMAL HEALTH?

We advise consumption of 4 mg of vitamin B_6 per day for men and women.

WHAT SPECIAL CIRCUMSTANCES MIGHT AFFECT THE AMOUNT OF VITAMIN B_6 YOU NEED TO TAKE?

You need to be particularly conscientious about taking the optimal dose of vitamin B_6 if you are pregnant or breast-feeding, take birth-control pills or certain medications, eat a high-protein diet, or consume large amounts of alcohol.

IS IT POSSIBLE TO CONSUME THE OPTIMAL AMOUNT OF VITAMIN B_6 THROUGH DIET ALONE?

While you could consume enough vitamin B_6 in your diet alone, few people in the United States meet even the RDAs for this vitamin, let alone our ODA. You may need to take a daily supplement to help you reach our recommended dose of 4 mg.

VITAMIN B$_{12}$—COBALAMIN

The history of vitamin B$_{12}$ dates back to the 19th century, when a ferocious form of anemia swept through parts of Europe. This disease was so fierce that it was often called *pernicious anemia*. No one was sure what caused it or how to treat it, but years later, it was finally determined that foods rich in B$_{12}$ could combat it. Today, because the B$_{12}$ molecule contains the trace element cobalt, some supplement labels list this vitamin as *cobalamin*. Like other B vitamins, vitamin B$_{12}$ is water-soluble.

History

When pernicious anemia was ravaging Europe, its symptoms were merciless—diarrhea and a sore mouth in the beginning and, often, severe mental disturbance and even death before long. Under the pressures of trying to understand this life-threatening disease, researchers frantically sought answers in a number of directions. Many, however, never seriously thought to blame a nutritional deficit. After all, they reasoned, victims of pernicious anemia appeared to be well nourished.

Finally, in the 1920s and 1930s, Nobel Prize–winning experimenters George Minot and William Murphy discovered clues to the disease. They demonstrated that patients who ate a lot of liver somehow recovered from this form of anemia. After many years of research, by the late 1940s, vitamin B$_{12}$ was isolated and identified as the substance that was so successful in overcoming the killer disease. Other foods contain B$_{12}$, too, but liver is one of the richest.

In order for your body to absorb the vitamin B_{12} that you consume, cells in the stomach lining must produce a protein called *intrinsic factor*. Without enough of this factor in the gastric juices, the intestines cannot absorb B_{12}, and a deficiency may occur.

Basic Functions

• Vitamin B_{12} is required for manufacturing and developing red blood cells in the marrow.

• Vitamin B_{12} is necessary for the body to use folic acid properly.

• Vitamin B_{12} is important in forming genetic material (nucleic acid) used by all cells.

• Vitamin B_{12} helps the nervous system function properly and is needed to produce the protective sheaths that cover the nerves.

• Vitamin B_{12} is involved in a number of chemical reactions important in carbohydrate, fat, and protein metabolism.

Signs of Deficiency

The disorder most often associated with a severe vitamin B_{12} deficiency is pernicious anemia. An individual who has this type of anemia may experience weakness, weight loss, pale skin, and psychological disturbances. Without prompt diagnosis and treatment of pernicious anemia, permanent nerve damage may occur. Blood and bone marrow cells may also change—specifically, abnormally large red blood cells may be released into the bloodstream.

A vitamin B_{12} deficiency may produce other disorders and symptoms as well, many of them related to the nervous system. Tingling in the hands or feet, trouble walking, moodiness, and depression are among the problems caused by B_{12} deficiency.

Even if you get enough vitamin B_{12} in your diet, you may develop a deficiency if your body does not absorb enough of the nutrient. If your stomach fails to manufacture sufficient quantities of intrinsic factor, you may not be able to use the B_{12} in your diet.

Some of the problems associated with a vitamin B_{12} deficiency are related to the close connection between B_{12} and folic acid, another B vitamin. Without adequate amounts of B_{12}, the body cannot process and use folic acid. Even if you consume plenty of folic acid, then, you can experience symptoms of a folic acid deficiency if you don't consume enough B_{12}.

Who's at Risk for Vitamin B_{12} Deficiency?

If you answer yes to any of the following questions, you have an above-average risk of developing a vitamin B_{12} deficiency.

• *Are you a strict vegetarian?* Vitamin B_{12} exists naturally only in animal foods and products. Children on vegetarian diets are particularly susceptible to deficiencies, because they have not yet built up stores of B_{12} in their liver.

• *Are you an older person?* Older people often have more trouble absorbing B_{12} than younger people do, because their bodies have more difficulty producing the intrinsic factor that enables them to absorb B_{12}.

• *Do you have tapeworms?* Although rare, tapeworms can cause a deficiency of vitamin B_{12}.

• *Are you taking medications such as colchicine (for gout), cholestyramine (for high cholesterol levels), or omeprazole (for ulcers)?* These medications interfere with absorption of vitamin B_{12}. Particular antibiotics, such as neomycin, can lower B_{12} levels, although scientists do not yet understand why.

• *Have parts of your stomach been surgically removed?* Intrinsic factor, which is important for absorption of B_{12}, is produced in the stomach.

• *Are you pregnant?* A fetus needs 0.1 to 0.2 mcg of vitamin B_{12} per day. According to the RDAs, pregnant women should consume an additional 0.2 mcg of vitamin B_{12} daily.

• *Are you breast-feeding?* A baby gets about 0.6 mcg of vitamin B_{12} per liter of breast milk. According to the RDAs, breast-feeding women should take an extra 0.6 mcg of B_{12} per day.

Toxicity

Toxicity has not been reported when people have consumed even large amounts of vitamin B_{12}.

Health Merits

Many statements have been made about vitamin B_{12}, most commonly that B_{12} can boost energy. Scientific evidence does not substantiate most of these claims, although research does show promise in the area of cardiovascular health.

CARDIOVASCULAR DISEASE

Vitamin B_{12} does appear to help prevent cardiovascular disease by decreasing levels of *homocysteine* (an amino acid that contributes to the risk of heart disease). One recent study found that three B

Recommended Dietary Allowances

Infants

0–6 months ....*0.3 mcg

6–12 months ....0.5 mcg

Children

1–3 years ....0.7 mcg

4–6 years ....1.0 mcg

7–10 years ....1.4 mcg

Male and Female Adolescents and Adults

11+ years ....2.0 mcg

Pregnant Women

....2.2 mcg

Lactating Women

.... 2.6 mcg

* A microgram is one-millionth of a gram; a milligram (in which many other vitamins are measured) is one-thousandth of a gram.

vitamins—B_{12}, B_6, and folic acid—were involved in the formation of homocysteine. When a person consumes little of these vitamins, the body produces high levels of homocysteine. Conversely, supplementation of these B vitamins appears to normalize homocysteine levels—and reduce the risk of heart disease.

• In 1993, researchers in South Africa studied 30 men with high levels of homocysteine and correspondingly low levels of vitamin B_{12}. The participants received varying amounts of B_{12} (as well as other B vitamins) or supplements of beta-carotene. Six weeks later, those who had received the B vitamin supplements had normal homocysteine levels. Those who did not take B vitamins still had elevated homocysteine—and thus a higher risk of cardiovascular disease.

How Much Vitamin B₁₂ Do You Need?

Your body needs little vitamin B_{12}. Consequently, RDAs are low—for example, only 2.0 mcg for adult men and women.

Optimal Daily Allowance

For you to achieve optimal health, we recommend taking 5 mcg of vitamin B_{12} per day—about two-and-a-half times the RDA. We think this is important because of the role that vitamin B_{12} plays in reducing levels of homocysteine, the amino acid that, in large amounts, may contribute to the development of cardiovascular disease.

Vitamin B₁₂ Content of Common Foods

Food Item	Amount of Vitamin (in mcg)
Anchovy (3 oz, raw)	0.53
Bacon (3 slices, fried)	0.33
Beef, bottom round (3½ oz, braised)	2.40
Beef, brisket (3½ oz, braised)	2.23
Beef soup, chunky (1 cup)	0.61

Beef, top round (3½ oz, broiled)..2.44
Blue cheese (1 oz) 0.35
Bologna, beef (1 slice)...0.33
Brie cheese (1 oz)..0.47
Camembert cheese (1 oz) 0.37
Carp (3 oz, raw)..1.30
Chicken, breast (½ breast, roasted)...0.32
Chicken, dark and light meat (3½ oz, roasted) 0.30
Chicken, leg (1, roasted) 0.35
Chicken soup, chunky (1 cup) 0.25
Clams (4 lg or 9 sm, raw)...42.03
Cod (3 oz, raw) 0.77
Corned beef (3½ oz, cooked)...1.63
Cottage cheese, low-fat (1 cup)..1.43
Crab (3 oz, cooked)...6.21
Egg (1 lg, boiled) 0.66
Flank steak (3½ oz, braised)..3.02
Ground beef, lean (3½ oz, baked)...1.77
Gruyere (1 oz) 0.45
Haddock (3 oz, raw)...1.02
Halibut (3 oz, raw) 1.01
Ham, canned (3½ oz) 0.78
Herring (3 oz, raw)...11.62
Hot dog, beef (1) 0.87

Food Sources

Foods of animal origin are excellent—and the only natural—sources of vitamin B_{12}. Meats (including liver and kidney), fish, poultry, milk, and cheese all contain this vitamin.

If you are a vegetarian, vitamin B_{12} supplements are probably a good choice. Soybean milk substitutes and breakfast cereals are often vitamin B_{12}-fortified.

Little vitamin B_{12} is lost in cooking. The vitamin is water-soluble but is very stable in the presence of heat.

Liver, beef (3½ oz, braised)..71.00
Liver, chicken (3½ oz, simmered).. 19.39
Mackerel (3 oz, raw) 7.40
Manhattan clam chowder (1 cup)..7.92
Milk, low-fat, 1% (8 oz)...0.90
Miso (½ cup) 0.29
Muenster cheese (1 oz) 0.42
Oysters (6 med, raw) 16.07
Pork, loin (3½ oz, roasted) 0.87
Pork, shoulder (3½ oz, roasted)...0.83
Provolone cheese (1 oz) 0.42
Ricotta cheese (½ cup)...0.36
Salmon (3 oz, raw) 2.70
Sardines, canned in oil (2)...2.15
Scallops (6 lg or 14 sm, raw) 1.30
Shrimp (12 lg, raw)...0.99
Swiss cheese (1 oz)...0.48
Swordfish (3 oz) 1.49
Trout (3 oz, raw) 6.62
Turkey, light and dark meat (3½ oz, roasted) 0.35
Yogurt, low-fat (8 oz) 1.28

How Much Vitamin B₁₂ Are People in the United States Getting?

According to government surveys in the mid-1980s, men tend to consume more vitamin B₁₂ than women do; men consumed 7.84 mcg per day, while women consumed 4.85 mcg. These averages are well above the RDAs of 2.0 mcg for both men and women.

How Much Vitamin B₁₂ Are You Getting?

Before you decide that you need to take vitamin supplements or change the way you eat, you should know where you stand and how much improvement you really need. To help you analyze your current diet, we've developed a system you can use to calculate your approximate vitamin B_{12} intake. (You'll find this system in the other vitamin and mineral chapters, too.) Following is a list of vitamin B_{12} food sources, arranged according to the percentage of our Optimal Daily Allowance of vitamin B_{12} contained in them. Since a 3 ounce serving of halibut contains 1.01 mcg of B_{12}—about one-fifth of the ODA—we've listed halibut in the 20 Percent category. (We have erred on the conservative side when rounding off percentages.)

To determine your average daily intake of vitamin B_{12}, start by keeping an accurate food diary for three or four days. The longer you keep the diary, the more accurate your calculations will be. Write down exactly what you eat and drink, together with an estimate of the serving size. Don't concern yourself with precisely how much B_{12} each food item contains; simply use the list to find the food item and the percentage of the ODA that it provides. Then add up all these percentages to see if you reach 100 percent each day.

If a particular item in your meals is missing from this list (it would be impossible for us to include every food item here), use the nutritional information on the food packaging. Most packaged foods are required to list their vitamin contents on the label.

After you've determined how much vitamin B_{12} you are obtaining from your diet each day, you can calculate whether you need to take supplements to reach the ODA. Let's say that you determine that you are getting 80 percent of your vitamin B_{12} target through diet alone. You are consuming 4 mcg of B_{12} in your diet (80 percent x 5 mcg = 4 mcg). To make up the difference, we would advise you to supplement your diet with 1 mcg of vitamin B_{12} in tablet form (5 mcg – 4 mcg = 1 mcg).

Virtually all multivitamin formulations will provide you with the extra B_{12} you need. (One popular brand contains 9 mcg of B_{12}.) Remember that no adverse effects have been reported with high doses of vitamin B_{12}, so you can consume doses even larger than the ODA to meet your needs without risk.

PERCENTAGE OF VITAMIN B$_{12}$ ODA

5 Percent

Bacon (3 slices, fried)
Blue cheese (1 oz)
Bologna, beef (1 slice)
Brie cheese (1 oz)
Chicken, breast (½, roasted)
Chicken, dark and light meat (3½ oz, roasted)
Chicken, leg (1, roasted)
Chicken soup, chunky (1 cup)
Gruyere (1 oz)
Miso (½ cup)
Muenster cheese (1 oz)
Provolone cheese (1 oz)
Ricotta cheese, part skim (1 oz)
Swiss cheese (1 oz)
Turkey, light and dark meat (3½ oz, roasted)

10 Percent

Anchovy (3 oz, raw)
Beef soup, chunky (1 cup)
Cod (3 oz, raw)
Egg (1 lg, boiled)
Ham, canned (3½ oz)
Hot dog, beef (1)
Milk, low-fat, 1% (8 oz)
Pork, loin (3½ oz, roasted)
Pork, shoulder (3½ oz, roasted)
Shrimp (12 lg, raw)

20 Percent

Carp (3 oz, raw)
Cottage cheese, low-fat (1 cup)
Haddock (3 oz, raw)
Halibut (3 oz, raw)

Scallops (6 lg or 14 sm, raw)
Swordfish (3 oz, raw)
Yogurt, low-fat (8 oz)

30 Percent

Bran Flakes cereal (1 oz)
Corn Flakes cereal (1 oz)
Corned beef (3½ oz, cooked)
Ground beef, lean (3½ oz, baked)
Raisin Bran cereal (1 oz)

40 Percent

Beef, bottom round (3½ oz, braised)
Beef, brisket (3½ oz, braised)
Beef, top round (3½ oz, broiled)
Sardines, canned in oil (2)

50 Percent

Salmon (3 oz, raw)

60 Percent

Flank steak (3½ oz, broiled)

100 Percent or More

Breakfast cereals, most (1 oz)
Clams (4 lg or 9 sm, raw)
Crab (3 oz, cooked)
Herring (3 oz, raw)
Liver, beef (3½ oz, braised)
Liver, chicken (3½ oz, simmered)
Mackerel (3 oz, raw)
Manhattan clam chowder (1 cup)
Oysters (6 med, raw)
Product 19 cereal (1 oz)
Total cereal (1 oz)
Trout (3 oz, raw)
Tuna, bluefin (3 oz, raw)

Our Recommendations

HOW MUCH VITAMIN B$_{12}$ DO YOU NEED TO ACHIEVE OPTIMAL HEALTH?

We advise consuming 5 mcg of vitamin B$_{12}$ per day, a level two-and-a-half times the RDA.

WHAT SPECIAL CIRCUMSTANCES MIGHT AFFECT THE AMOUNT OF VITAMIN B$_{12}$ YOU NEED TO TAKE?

You need to be especially conscientious about taking optimal doses of vitamin B$_{12}$ if you are an older person; are a strict vegetarian; are pregnant or breast-feeding; have had stomach surgery; take certain medications for gout, high cholesterol, or ulcers; or have tapeworms.

IS IT POSSIBLE TO CONSUME THE OPTIMAL AMOUNT OF VITAMIN B$_{12}$ THROUGH DIET ALONE?

In fact, many people do consume the optimal amount of vitamin B$_{12}$ through diet. Men consume an average of 7.84 mcg of vitamin B$_{12}$ per day, which is more than 50 percent higher than our ODA. The average B$_{12}$ intake of women (4.85 mcg) is only slightly below our ODA.

OTHER B VITAMINS

In addition to niacin, vitamins B_6 and B_{12}, and folic acid—vitamins described in individual chapters—there are B vitamins that receive less attention but that are also essential to health and well-being. True, these other Bs may not hold the promise of preventing birth defects (as folic acid does) or of reducing blood cholesterol levels (as niacin does), but they are still important. All are essential, water-soluble nutrients.

VITAMIN B_1: THIAMIN

Thiamin, the first of the B vitamins to be discovered, was initially isolated in the mid-1920s. Today we know that thiamin plays an important part in changing energy stored in carbohydrates to a form that our bodies can use. Thiamin is also necessary for the nervous system to function properly, and it may be involved with producing nerve transmitters.

Signs of Deficiency

The first symptoms of a thiamin deficiency can include constipation, fatigue, and loss of appetite. Probably the best-known thiamin deficiency disorder—a disease called beriberi—occurs in the most severe cases of deprivation.

Beriberi was rampant in parts of Asia in the 19th century, afflicting rice-consuming people at a time when mills produced highly polished, refined rice. This processing removed the thiamin-rich husks, and the diets and health of millions of people suffered. Symptoms of beriberi vary depending on age, duration of the deficiency, and other factors, but among the most common signs are loss of muscle strength, leg spasms or paralysis, mental confusion, and depression.

While beriberi has been reported in the United States, it is rare in this country. Thiamin supplements in many cereals and the wide availability of other thiamin-containing foods have kept out the disease here. Even so, beriberi is sometimes seen in alcoholics,

Who's at Risk for Thiamin Deficiency?

If you answer yes to any of the following questions, you have an above-average risk of developing a thiamin deficiency.

• *Do you have diabetes?* This condition can increase the amount of thiamin excreted in the urine.

• *Do you have a disorder that increases your metabolic rate?* Such disorders—including infections, fevers, hyperactivity, and hyperthyroidism—increase thiamin requirements.

• *Do you consume large amounts of alcohol?* Alcohol interferes with the absorption of thiamin, and alcoholics tend to have poor diets that may be deficient in thiamin.

• *Do you eat large amounts of raw fish?* An enzyme called thiaminase, found in raw fish, inactivates thiamin; cooking, however, destroys this enzyme.

• *Do you consume large amounts of carbohydrates?* Your body needs thiamin to metabolize carbohydrates. The more carbohydrates you consume, therefore, the more thiamin you require.

• *Are you pregnant or breast-feeding?* According to the RDAs, women should take an additional .4 mg of thiamin per day during pregnancy to accommodate for their own increased needs and for the growth of the fetus. Women who are breast-feeding should take an additional .5 mg of thiamin per day to compensate for the amount of the vitamin lost in breast milk.

because their diets are poor and because alcohol interferes with thiamin absorption.

Toxicity

Even with large oral doses of thiamin, no toxic effects have been reported. High doses administered intravenously, however, have produced severe allergic reactions (anaphylactic shock).

Optimal Daily Allowance

We believe that the optimal intake of thiamin, based on its role in the body, is 1.5 mg per day. This dose approximates the highest RDA. No one should require more thiamin than this.

Recommended Dietary Allowances

Infants

0–6 months	0.3 mg
6–12 months	0.4 mg

Children

1–3 years	0.7 mg
4–6 years	0.9 mg
7–10 years	1.0 mg

Male Adolescents and Adults

11–14 years	1.3 mg
15–50 years	1.5 mg
51+ years	1.2 mg

Female Adolescents and Adults

11–50 years	1.1 mg
51+ years	1.0 mg

Pregnant Women

	1.5 mg

Lactating Women

	1.6 mg

Thiamin Content of Common Foods

Food Item	*Amount of Vitamin (in mg)*
Acorn squash (½ cup, baked)	0.17
Avocado, California (½ med)	0.10
Avocado, Florida (½ med)	0.16
Bacon (3 slices, fried)	0.13
Bagel (1)	0.21
Baker's yeast (1 oz, dry)	0.66
Beef, top round (3½ oz, broiled)	0.11
Black beans (1 cup, boiled)	0.42
Blackeye peas (1 cup, boiled)	0.35
Brazil nuts (1 oz)	0.28
Brewer's yeast (1 oz)	4.43
Broadbeans (1 cup, boiled)	0.17
Carrot juice, canned (6 oz)	0.17
Corn, yellow (½ cup, boiled)	0.18
Ham, canned (3½ oz)	0.96
Hazelnuts (1 oz)	0.14
Kidney beans (1 cup, boiled)	0.28
Leg of lamb (3 oz, roasted)	0.13
Lentils (1 cup, boiled)	0.34
Lima beans (1 cup, boiled)	0.30
Liver, chicken (3½ oz, simmered)	0.15
Liver, beef (3½ oz, braised)	0.20

Food Sources

Thiamin is present in many foods. Some of the best sources include whole-grain or enriched breads and cereals, brewer's yeast, liver and other organ meats, lean cuts of pork, peas, beans, and nuts and seeds.

Heat or immersion of foods in water during cooking can destroy thiamin. To retain this water-soluble vitamin, cook thiamin-containing foods in only small amounts of water.

Macadamia nuts (1 oz)..0.10
Mackerel (3 oz, raw)...0.15
Mango (1 med)..0.12
Marinara sauce (1 cup)...0.11
Miso (½ cup)...0.13
Navy beans (1 cup, boiled)...0.37
Oatmeal, instant (1 pkt)..0.53
Orange (1 med)...0.12
Orange juice, from concentrate (8 oz)...0.20
Peanuts (1 oz)...0.19
Peas (½ cup, boiled)...0.21
Pecans (1 oz)...0.24
Pineapple juice, canned (8 oz)..0.14
Pinto beans (1 cup, boiled)...0.32
Pistachio nuts (1 oz)..0.23
Pork, loin (3½ oz, roasted)...0.61
Pork, shoulder (3½ oz, roasted)..0.54
Potato (baked, with skin)...0.22
Potato (baked, without skin)...0.16
Rice, brown (1 cup, cooked)...0.18
Rice, white, enriched (1 cup, cooked)..0.23
Salmon (3 oz, raw)..0.19
Spaghetti, enriched (1 cup, cooked)..0.20
Sunflower seeds (1 oz, dried)..0.65
Tofu (½ cup, raw)..0.10
Trout (3 oz, raw)...0.30
Wheat germ (¼ cup, toasted)..0.47
White bread (1 slice)..0.11
Whole-wheat bread (1 slice)...0.09
Yogurt, low-fat (8 oz)..0.10

How Much Thiamin Are People in the United States Getting?

Surveys in the mid-1980s showed that adult men consumed an average of 1.75 mg of thiamin per day; women averaged 1.05 mg per day. While these figures confirm that the average male gets more thiamin than the ODA, and that the average female comes close to the ODA, many people fall significantly below the average.

How Much Thiamin Are You Getting?

Use the information in this section and in similar sections for the other B vitamins in this chapter to calculate the amount of a particular vitamin you are getting in your diet. Following is a list of common food sources of the vitamin (thiamin, in this case), arranged according to the percentage of our Optimal Daily Allowance of the vitamin contained in them.

To determine your average daily intake of thiamin (and the other B vitamins in this chapter), start by keeping an accurate food diary for three or four days. Write down exactly what you eat and drink, together with an estimate of the serving size. Find the food item on the chart, and determine the percentage of the ODA that it provides. Then add up all these percentages to see if you reach 100 percent each day.

If a particular item in your meals is missing from the chart, use the nutritional information on the food packaging. Most packaged foods are required to list their vitamin contents on the label.

After you've determined how much of the vitamin you are obtaining from your diet each day, you can calculate whether you need to take supplements to reach the ODA. Let's say that you determine that you are getting 60 percent of your thiamin target through diet alone. You are consuming 0.9 mg of thiamin in your diet (60 percent x 1.5 mg = 0.9 mg). To make up the difference, we would advise you to supplement your diet with 0.6 mg of thiamin in tablet form (1.5 mg – 0.9 mg = 0.6 mg). Most multivitamins contain at least the ODA for thiamin, and often more—so if you take a multivitamin tablet each day, you're probably getting all the extra thiamin you need without any real risk.

PERCENTAGE OF THIAMIN ODA
5 Percent

Avocado, California (½ med)
Bacon (3 slices, fried)
Beef, top round (3½ oz, broiled)
Figs (10, dried)
Flank steak (3½ oz, broiled)
Grapefruit juice (8 oz)
Hazelnuts (1 oz)
Leg of lamb (3 oz, roasted)
Macadamia nuts (1 oz)
Mango (1 med)
Marinara sauce (1 cup)
Milk, low-fat, 1% (8 oz)
Miso (½ cup)
Orange (1 med)
Pineapple juice, canned (8 oz)
Tofu (½ cup, raw)
White or wheat bread (1 slice)
Yogurt, low-fat (8 oz)

10 Percent

Acorn squash (½ cup, baked)
Avocado, Florida (½ med)
Bagel (1)
Brazil nuts (1 oz)
Broadbeans (1 cup, boiled)
Carrot juice, canned (6 oz)
Corn, yellow (½ cup, boiled)
Corn tortilla (1)
Garbanzo beans (1 cup, boiled)
Great Northern beans (1 cup, boiled)
Kidney beans (1 cup, boiled)
Liver, beef (3½ oz, braised)
Liver, chicken (3½ oz, simmered)
Mackerel (3 oz, raw)

Orange juice, from concentrate (8 oz)
Peanuts (1 oz)
Peas (½ cup, boiled)
Pecans (1 oz)
Pistachio nuts (1 oz)
Potato (baked, without skin)
Rice, brown (1 cup, cooked)
Rice, white, enriched (1 cup, cooked)
Salmon (3 oz, raw)
Spaghetti, enriched (1 cup, cooked)

20 Percent

Black beans (1 cup, boiled)
Blackeye peas (1 cup, boiled)
Bran Flakes cereal (1 oz)
Corn Flakes cereal (1 oz)
Cream of Wheat, instant (1 pkt)
Lentils (1 cup, boiled)
Lima beans (1 cup, boiled)
Navy beans (1 cup, boiled)
Pinto beans (1 cup, boiled)
Raisin Bran cereal (1 oz)
Trout (3 oz, raw)

30 Percent

Oatmeal, instant (1 pkt)
Pork, shoulder (3½ oz, roasted)
Wheat germ (¼ cup, toasted)

40 Percent

Baker's yeast (1 oz, dry)
Pork, loin (3½ oz, roasted)
Sunflower seeds (1 oz, dried)

60 Percent

Ham, canned (3½ oz)

---
100 Percent or More

Breakfast cereals, most (1 oz)
Brewer's yeast (1 oz)
Product 19 cereal (1 oz)
Total cereal (1 oz)

Our Recommendations

HOW MUCH THIAMIN DO YOU NEED TO ACHIEVE OPTIMAL HEALTH?

We recommend that you consume 1.5 mg of thiamin per day.

WHAT SPECIAL CIRCUMSTANCES MIGHT AFFECT THE AMOUNT OF THIAMIN YOU NEED TO TAKE?

If you have diabetes or a metabolic disorder, eat lots of carbohydrates or raw fish, consume large amounts of alcohol, or are pregnant or breast-feeding, you need to be particularly conscientious about consuming the ODA for thiamin.

IS IT POSSIBLE TO CONSUME THE OPTIMAL AMOUNT OF THIAMIN THROUGH DIET ALONE?

Many people in the United States come close to reaching or actually do reach the ODA for thiamin solely through diet. If you are not one of these people, you can get supplemental thiamin easily as part of multivitamin or B-complex preparations.

VITAMIN B_2: RIBOFLAVIN

Toward the end of the 19th century, a fluorescent pigment was detected in milk whey; subsequently, the pigment was found in other sources (liver and eggs) as well. Although its significance was not initially understood, we in the 20th century have come to appreciate its growth-promoting properties. In the 1930s, the nutrient was isolated and identified. It was vitamin B_2, or riboflavin.

Riboflavin is important to the complex processes in your body that give you energy from the foods you consume. It is also needed to convert tryptophan to niacin.

Signs of Deficiency

Studies have shown that signs of deficiency can occur with a consumption of riboflavin at 0.55 mg per day or less. These signs won't occur overnight, however, because your kidney and liver store small amounts of B_2, thus postponing deficiency symptoms for some three to four months of deprivation.

The initial signs of riboflavin deficiency tend to be general in nature, including such things as lost appetite and impaired growth. Soon after, local problems can appear, such as sores and cracks on the nose, lips, and corners of the mouth; tongue swelling and loss of the sense of taste; scaly skin; anemia; reddened eyes and

Who's at Risk for Riboflavin Deficiency?

If you answer yes to any of the following questions, you have an above-average risk of developing a riboflavin deficiency.

• *Do you chronically take medications such as diuretics, phobenicid (an antigout drug), or antidepressants (tricyclics)?* Diuretics and phobenicid increase the excretion of riboflavin in the urine; antidepressants interfere with the metabolism of riboflavin.

• *Do you have diabetes?* Diabetics tend to excrete increased amounts of riboflavin in their urine.

• *Do you exercise, even moderately?* As you expend energy, you use riboflavin more rapidly.

• *Are you pregnant or breast-feeding?* The RDAs advise taking an additional .3 mg of riboflavin per day during pregnancy, an additional .5 mg per day during the first six months of breast-feeding, and an additional .4 mg for longer periods of breast-feeding.

dimmed vision; and depression or hysteria (as a result of damage to the nervous tissue).

Because riboflavin is necessary for vitamin B_6 and niacin to work in the body, a B_2 deficiency can also produce symptoms related to shortages of these other B vitamins. (Refer to chapters on vitamin B_6 and niacin for information about the signs of these deficiencies.)

Toxicity

Taking excessive amounts of riboflavin has no known adverse effects.

Recommended Dietary Allowances

Infants

0–6 months	0.4 mg
6–12 months	0.5 mg

Children

1–3 years	0.8 mg
4–6 years	1.1 mg
7–10 years	1.2 mg

Male Adolescents and Adults

11–14 years	1.5 mg
15–18 years	1.8 mg
19–50 years	1.7 mg
51+ years	1.4 mg

Female Adolescents and Adults

11–50 years	1.3 mg
51+ years	1.2 mg

Pregnant Women

	1.6 mg

Lactating Women

first 6 months	1.8 mg
second 6 months	1.7 mg

How Much Riboflavin Do You Need?

Because your body stores only small amounts of riboflavin that can gradually become depleted, you need to replenish this B vitamin regularly.

Optimal Daily Allowance

We recommend an Optimal Daily Allowance of 1.8 mg of riboflavin per day, which corresponds to the highest RDA for this vitamin. We have seen no evidence to suggest that doses higher than 1.8 mg are necessary or optimal.

Riboflavin Content of Common Foods

Food Item	*Amount of Vitamin (in mg)*
Almonds (1 oz)	0.22
American cheese (1 oz)	0.10
Anchovy (3 oz, raw)	0.22
Apple (10 rings, dried)	0.10
Asparagus (6 spears, boiled)	0.11
Avocado, California (½ med)	0.10
Avocado, Florida (½ med)	0.18
Bagel (1)	0.16
Baker's yeast (1 oz)	1.53
Beef, bottom round (3½ oz, braised)	0.25
Beef, brisket (3½ oz, braised)	0.17
Beef soup, chunky (1 cup)	0.15
Beef, top round (3½ oz, broiled)	0.26
Beet greens (½ cup, boiled)	0.21
Black beans (1 cup, boiled)	0.10
Blue cheese (1 oz)	0.11
Brewer's yeast (1 oz)	1.21
Brie cheese (1 oz)	0.15
Broadbeans (1 cup, boiled)	0.15
Broccoli (½ cup, boiled)	0.16

Buttermilk (8 oz) 0.38
Cheddar cheese (1 oz) 0.11
Chicken, breast (½, roasted) 0.12
Chicken, dark and light meat (3½ oz, roasted)..............................0.17
Chicken, dark meat (3½ oz, roasted)...0.21
Chicken, leg (1, roasted)..0.20
Chicken, light meat (3½ oz, roasted)...0.12
Chicken soup, chunky (1 cup) 0.17
Chicken, thigh (1, roasted) 0.13
Chicken, wing (1, roasted).. 0.12
Clams (4 lg or 9 sm)..0.18
Colby cheese (1 oz) 0.11
Corned beef (3½ oz, cooked)..0.17
Cottage cheese, low-fat (8 oz) 0.37
Cream of Wheat, instant (1 pkt)..0.10
Egg (1 lg, boiled) 0.14
Figs (10, dried)..0.17
Flank steak (3½ oz, braised) 0.18
Garbanzo beans (1 cup, boiled) 0.10
Gouda cheese (1 oz)..0.10
Great Northern beans (1 cup, boiled) 0.10
Ground beef, lean (3½ oz, baked)..0.19
Ham (3½ oz, canned)..0.23

Food Sources

Generous amounts of riboflavin are available in milk and other
dairy foods, including cheese, ice cream, and yogurt. (The higher
the fat content of a dairy food, the less riboflavin it has.) Meats
(especially liver and other organ meats) and fish (including salmon
and tuna) are also good sources of riboflavin, as are enriched grain
products and green leafy vegetables such as broccoli and spinach.

Exposure to sunlight and ultraviolet light can destroy riboflavin.
It is important, therefore, to store riboflavin-rich foods in refriger-
ators, cupboards, and/or opaque containers that guard them
from sunlight.

Herring (3 oz, raw) 0.20
Ice cream, vanilla (1 cup) 0.33
Ice milk, vanilla (1 cup)...0.35
Kidney beans (1 cup, boiled)...0.10
Lamb, loin chop (1, boiled)...0.16
Lamb, rib chop (1, boiled)...0.14
Leg of lamb (3 oz, roasted) 0.23
Lima beans (1 cup, boiled) 0.10
Limburger cheese (1 oz)...0.14
Liver, beef (3½ oz, braised)..4.10
Liver, chicken (3½ oz, simmered) 1.75
Mackerel (3 oz, raw) 0.27
Marinara sauce (1 cup)..0.15
Milk, low-fat, 1% (8 oz)..0.41
Miso (½ cup) 0.35
Monterey cheese (1 oz)...0.11
Mushrooms (½ cup, raw)..0.16
Navy beans (1 cup, boiled)..0.11
Oatmeal, instant (1 pkt) 0.29
Oysters (6 med, raw)..0.14
Peaches (10 halves, dried) 0.28
Pears (10 halves, dried)...0.25
Peas (½ cup, boiled)...0.12
Pinto beans (1 cup, boiled) 0.16
Pork, loin (3½ oz, roasted) 0.32
Pork, shoulder (3½ oz, roasted) 0.32
Prune juice, canned (8 oz)..0.18
Prunes (10, dried)...0.14
Pudding, vanilla, homemade (1 cup) 0.41
Raisins, golden seedless (⅔ cup)...0.19
Ricotta cheese, part skim (½ cup) 0.23
Salmon (3 oz, raw)...0.32
Sweet potato (1 med, baked)..0.15
Swiss cheese (1 oz)...0.10
Trout (3 oz, raw)...0.28
Turkey, dark meat (3½ oz, roasted) 0.24

Turkey, dark and light meat (3½ oz, roasted) 0.18
Turkey, light meat (3½ oz, roasted) 0.13
Wheat germ (¼ cup, toasted) 0.23
Yogurt, low-fat (8 oz)..0.40

How Much Riboflavin Are People in the United States Getting

U.S. Department of Agriculture surveys show that men take an average of 2.08 mg of riboflavin per day; women average 1.34 mg. According to these surveys, most people appear to be meeting their daily needs through diet. Because these figures are averages, however, they also suggest that many people probably take significantly less B_2 than they should.

How Much Riboflavin Are You Getting?

To determine whether you are reaching the ODA of riboflavin, use the information from the following list. For an explanation, refer back to "How Much Thiamin Are You Getting?" earlier in this chapter.

PERCENTAGE OF RIBOFLAVIN ODA
5 Percent

American cheese (1 oz)
Apple (10 rings, dried)
Asparagus (6 spears, boiled)
Avocado, California (½ med)
Bagel (1)
Beef, brisket (3½ oz, braised)
Beef soup, chunky (1 cup)
Black beans (1 cup, boiled)
Blue cheese (1 oz)
Brie cheese (1 oz)
Broadbeans (1 cup, boiled)
Broccoli (½ cup, boiled)

Cheddar cheese (1 oz)
Chicken, breast (½, roasted)
Chicken, dark and light meat (3½ oz, roasted)
Chicken, light meat (3½ oz, roasted)
Chicken, thigh (1, roasted)
Chicken, wing (1, roasted)
Chicken soup, chunky (1 cup)
Colby cheese (1 oz)
Corned beef (3½ oz, cooked)
Cream of Wheat, instant (1 pkt)
Egg (1 lg, boiled)
Figs (10, dried)
Garbanzo beans (1 cup, boiled)
Gouda cheese (1 oz)
Great Northern beans (1 cup, boiled)
Kidney beans (1 cup, boiled)
Lamb, loin chop (1, broiled)
Lamb, rib chop (1, broiled)
Lima beans (1 cup, boiled)
Limberger cheese (1 oz)
Marinara sauce (1 cup)
Monterey cheese (1 oz)
Mushrooms (½ cup, raw)
Navy beans (1 cup, boiled)
Oysters (6 med, raw)
Peas (½ cup, boiled)
Pinto beans (1 cup, boiled)
Prunes (10, dried)
Sweet potato (1 med, baked)
Swiss cheese (1 oz)
Turkey, light meat (3½ oz, roasted)

10 Percent

Almonds (1 oz)
Anchovy (3 oz, raw)
Avocado, Florida (½, med)
Beef, bottom round (3½ oz, braised)

Beef, top round (3½ oz, braised)
Beet greens (½ cup, boiled)
Chicken, dark meat (3½ oz, roasted)
Chicken, leg (1, roasted)
Clams (4 lg or 9 sm)
Flank steak (3½ oz, broiled)
Ground beef, lean (3½ oz, baked)
Ham, canned (3½ oz)
Herring (3 oz, raw)
Ice cream, vanilla (1 cup)
Ice milk, vanilla (1 cup)
Leg of lamb (3 oz, roasted)
Mackerel (3 oz, raw)
Miso (½ cup)
Oatmeal, instant (1 pkt)
Peach (10 halves, dried)
Pear (10 halves, dried)
Pork, loin (3½ oz, roasted)
Pork, shoulder (3½ oz, roasted)
Prune juice, canned (8 oz)
Ricotta cheese, part skim (½ cup)
Salmon (3 oz, raw)
Trout (3 oz, raw)
Turkey, dark and light meat (3½ oz, roasted)
Turkey, dark meat (3½ oz, roasted)
Wheat germ (¼ cup, toasted)

20 Percent

Bran Flakes cereal (1 oz)
Buttermilk (8 oz)
Corn Flakes cereal (1 oz)
Cottage cheese, low-fat (8 oz)
Milk, low-fat, 1% (8 oz)
Pudding, vanilla, homemade (1 cup)
Raisin Bran cereal (1 oz)
Yogurt, low-fat (8 oz)

70 Percent
Brewer's yeast (1 oz)

90 Percent
Baker's yeast (1 oz, dry)
Breakfast cereals, most (1 oz)
Liver, chicken (3½ oz, simmered)
Product 19 cereal (1 oz)
Total cereal (1 oz)

100 Percent or More
Liver, beef (3½ oz, braised)

Our Recommendations

HOW MUCH RIBOFLAVIN DO YOU NEED TO ACHIEVE OPTIMAL HEALTH?

We recommend an optimal intake of 1.8 mg of riboflavin per day. No evidence indicates that you need more.

WHAT SPECIAL CIRCUMSTANCES MIGHT AFFECT THE AMOUNT OF RIBOFLAVIN YOU NEED TO TAKE?

If you have diabetes, if you exercise, if you take certain medications (including diuretics or tricyclic antidepressants), or if you are pregnant or breast-feeding, be particularly conscientious about getting your ODA for riboflavin.

IS IT POSSIBLE TO CONSUME THE OPTIMAL AMOUNT OF RIBOFLAVIN THROUGH DIET ALONE?

Surveys show that, on average, men do consume their ODA of riboflavin through diet, and women tend to come close. These are averages, however; many people actually fall short and need a multivitamin supplement or B-complex tablet to help them get an optimal level of riboflavin.

PANTOTHENIC ACID

Pantothenic acid gets its name from the Greek word *pantos*, which means "everywhere." That's an indication of just how prevalent this B vitamin is in plants and animals. At least a small amount of pantothenic acid is present in most of the foods we eat.

Once you consume pantothenic acid, your body changes most of this B vitamin into a substance called *coenzyme* A, which is required to convert carbohydrates, fats, and some proteins into energy. Pantothenic acid is also necessary for the body to produce hormones and to form hemoglobin and a neurotransmitter called *acetylcholine*.

Signs of Deficiency

All foods contain at least some pantothenic acid, and since the body needs only limited amounts of this nutrient, the risks of a deficiency are small. In general, people who do experience this deficiency are deficient in all of the B vitamins.

Because pantothenic acid deficiency is so rare, diseases specifically caused by it have not been clearly identified—with one possible exception. During the 1940s, prisoners of war in the Far East

---

Who's at Risk for Pantothenic Acid Deficiency?

If you answer yes to any of the following questions, you have an above-average risk of developing a pantothenic acid deficiency.

• *Does your diet consist largely of highly processed foods?* Processing tends to deplete the amount of pantothenic acid in foods.

• *Do you have diabetes?* This disease seems to alter metabolism and increase the excretion of pantothenic acid.

• *Do you drink large amounts of alcohol?* Chronic and excessive use of alcohol can lead to a decrease in the pantothenic acid in your tissues.

---

developed severe pain, numbness, and tingling in their feet and toes. Their condition was given the name *burning foot syndrome*. Symptoms improved when the prisoners were given pantothenic acid but did not respond positively when they took other B vitamins. These men were severely malnourished and deficient in all vitamins, however, not just in B vitamins. So while their condition seemed to get better with administration of pantothenic acid, studies were never conducted to determine whether lack of this B vitamin was indeed responsible for the illness.

In laboratory experiments, scientists have deprived humans of this B vitamin for long periods of time. In this situation, the most commonly produced symptoms were headaches, nausea, abdominal cramps, fatigue, depression, increased susceptibility to colds, insomnia, and numbness and tingling in the hands and feet.

Toxicity

The human body excretes excessive amounts of pantothenic acid in urine. Not surprisingly, then, serious signs of toxicity have not been reported, although very high doses (10 g or more per day) occasionally produce diarrhea or water retention.

Health Merits

Pantothenic acid has no proven uses for treating disease. Although some faddists have claimed that this B vitamin can improve the condition of people with rheumatoid arthritis, scientific proof does not exist to support this claim.

How Much Pantothenic Acid Do You Need?

You can't count on the RDAs to guide you here. Formal RDAs have not been established for pantothenic acid. Studies indicate that daily doses of 4 to 7 mg are sufficient to meet the needs of adults, including pregnant and lactating women.

Optimal Daily Allowance

Upon reviewing the existing research, we have concluded that an optimal intake of pantothenic acid in the range of 4 to 7 mg should be sufficient for adults, including pregnant and breast-feeding women. Because there are no known safety concerns for this vitamin, we recommend that you take the high end of the range (7 mg).

Pantothenic Acid Content of Common Foods

Food Item	Amount of Vitamin (in mg)
Acorn squash (½ cup, baked)	0.51
Avocado, California (½ med)	0.84
Avocado, Florida (½ med)	1.47
Beef, bottom round (3½ oz, braised)	0.40
Beef, top round (3½ oz, broiled)	0.48
Black beans (1 cup, boiled)	0.42
Blackeye peas (1 cup, boiled)	0.70
Buttermilk (8 oz)	0.67
Butternut squash (½ cup, boiled)	0.37
Carrot juice, canned (6 oz)	0.42
Cashews (1 oz)	0.35
Chicken, breast (½, roasted)	0.92
Chicken, dark and light meat (3½ oz, roasted)	1.03
Chicken, leg (1, roasted)	1.32
Chicken, thigh (1, roasted)	0.69
Corn (½ cup, boiled)	0.72
Corned beef (3½ oz, cooked)	0.42

Food Sources

Organ meats, salmon, legumes, whole-grain cereals, eggs, and yeast are among the best sources of pantothenic acid. At least some pantothenic acid is present in most foods, however, including chicken, milk, and numerous fruits and vegetables.

Cottage cheese, low-fat (1 cup)..0.49
Dates (10, dried)...0.65
Egg (1 lg, boiled) 0.86
Figs (10, dried) 0.81
Flank steak (3½ oz, broiled) 0.44
Garbanzo beans (1 cup, boiled) 0.47
Grapefruit (½ med)..0.35
Great Northern beans (1 cup, boiled) 0.47
Ham, canned (3½ oz) 0.39
Herring (3 oz, raw)...0.55
Hubbard squash (½ cup, baked)...0.46
Ice cream, vanilla (1 cup)..0.65
Ice milk, vanilla (1 cup) 0.66
Kidney beans (1 cup, boiled)..0.39
Lentils (1 cup, boiled) 1.26
Lima beans (1 cup, boiled)...0.79
Liver, beef (3½ oz, braised)...4.57
Liver, chicken (3½ oz, simmered)..5.41
Mackerel (3 oz, raw) 0.73
Milk, low-fat, 1% (8 oz)...0.79
Miso (½ cup)..0.36
Mushrooms (½ cup, raw) 0.77
Navy beans (1 cup, boiled) 0.46
Oatmeal, instant (1 pkt) 0.35
Orange (1 med) 0.35
Orange juice, from concentrate (8 oz).....................................0.39
Parsnips (½ cup, boiled) 0.46
Peanuts (1 oz)...0.79
Pecans (1 oz)..0.49
Pork loin (3½ oz, roasted) 0.55
Pork, shoulder (3½ oz, roasted)...0.50
Potato (baked, without skin) 0.87
Potato (baked, with skin)...1.12
Prunes (10, dried) 0.39
Salmon (3 oz, raw) 1.41
Strawberries (1 cup, fresh)...0.51

Sweet potato (1 med, baked) 0.74
Swordfish (3 oz, raw) 0.35
Tomato juice (6 oz)..0.46
Trout (3 oz, raw) 1.65
Turkey, dark and light meat (3½ oz, roasted) 0.86
Wheat germ (¼ cup, toasted)..0.39
Yogurt, low-fat (8 oz) 1.34

How Much Pantothenic Acid Are People in the United States Getting?

Studies have shown that people in the United States consume an average of 5 to 10 mg of pantothenic acid per day; some people get up to 16 mg. Deficiencies of this vitamin are unlikely except in people who maintain severely restrictive or unusual diets for long periods of time.

How Much Pantothenic Acid Are You Getting?

To determine whether you are reaching the ODA of pantothenic acid, use the information from the following list. For an explanation, refer back to "How Much Thiamin Are You Getting?" earlier in this chapter.

PERCENTAGE OF PANTOTHENIC ACID ODA
5 Percent

Acorn squash (½ cup, baked)
Beef, bottom round (3½ oz, braised)
Beef, top round (3½ oz, broiled)
Black beans (1 cup, boiled)
Buttermilk (8 oz)
Butternut squash (½ cup, boiled)
Carrot juice, canned (6 oz)
Cashews (1 oz)
Chicken, thigh (1, roasted)

Corned beef (3½ oz, cooked)
Cottage cheese, low-fat (1 cup)
Dates (10, dried)
Flank steak (3½ oz, broiled)
Garbanzo beans (1 cup, boiled)
Grapefruit (½ med)
Great Northern beans (1 cup, boiled)
Ham, canned (3½ oz)
Herring (3 oz, raw)
Hubbard squash (½ cup, baked)
Ice cream, vanilla (1 cup)
Ice milk, vanilla (1 cup)
Kidney beans (1 cup, boiled)
Miso (½ cup)
Navy beans (1 cup, boiled)
Oatmeal, instant (1 pkt)
Orange (1 med)
Orange juice, from concentrate (8 oz)
Parsnips (½ cup, boiled)
Pecans (1 oz)
Pinto beans (1 cup, boiled)
Pork, loin (3½ oz, roasted)
Pork, shoulder (3½ oz, roasted)
Prunes (10, dried)
Strawberries (1 cup, fresh)
Swordfish (3 oz, raw)
Tomato juice (6 oz)
Wheat germ (¼ cup, toasted)

10 Percent

Avocado, California (½ med)
Blackeye peas (1 cup, boiled)
Chicken, breast (½, roasted)
Chicken, dark and light meat (3½ oz, roasted)
Chicken, leg (1, roasted)
Corn (½ cup, boiled)

Egg (1 lg, boiled)
Figs (10, dried)
Lentils (1 cup, boiled)
Lima beans (1 cup, boiled)
Milk, low-fat, 1% (8 oz)
Mushrooms (½ cup, raw)
Peanuts (1 oz)
Potato (baked, with skin)
Potato (baked, without skin)
Sweet potato (1 med, baked)
Turkey, dark and light meat (3½ oz, roasted)
Yogurt, low-fat (8 oz)

20 Percent

Avocado, Florida (½ med)
Salmon (3 oz, raw)
Trout (3 oz, raw)

60 Percent

Liver, beef (3½ oz, braised)

70 Percent

Liver, chicken (3½ oz, simmered)

Our Recommendations

HOW MUCH PANTOTHENIC ACID DO YOU NEED TO ACHIEVE OPTIMAL HEALTH?

We recommend an optimal range of 4 to 7 mg of pantothenic acid per day. Since no toxicity risks are associated with this vitamin, most people can take the high end of the range (7 mg) without concern.

WHAT SPECIAL CIRCUMSTANCES MIGHT AFFECT THE AMOUNT OF PANTOTHENIC ACID YOU NEED TO TAKE?

If you eat a lot of processed foods, drink large amounts of alcohol, or have diabetes, be certain to consume the ODA of pantothenic acid regularly.

IS IT POSSIBLE TO CONSUME THE OPTIMAL AMOUNT OF PANTOTHENIC ACID THROUGH DIET ALONE?

Most people in the United States consume 5 to 10 mg of pantothenic acid—within the ODA range—in their diets each day. If you get less than the ODA, however, you can meet your needs by taking multivitamin tablets or B-complex supplements.

BIOTIN

Biotin gets its name from the Greek word *bios*, meaning "life." Bacteria in the human intestines seem to produce enough biotin to meet the body's needs. This B vitamin is also available in common foods—most notably in organ meats.

Biotin is important in a number of processes, including the body's manufacturing and use of fats, carbohydrates, and proteins.

Signs of Deficiency

Biotin deficiencies are rare. People who do have them complain of dry and scaly skin, which is typically followed by loss of appetite,

Who's at Risk for Biotin Deficiency?

If you answer yes to any of the following questions, you have an above-average risk of developing a biotin deficiency.

• *Do you consume large amounts of raw egg whites?* Egg whites contain an undigestible protein, avidin, which interferes with the body's absorption of biotin. Cooking eggs, however, destroys this protein.

• *Are you pregnant?* Levels of biotin in the blood of pregnant women tend to be lower than levels in nonpregnant women.

• *Are you breast-feeding?* Because biotin is excreted in breast milk, lactating mothers may need to consume more biotin.

• *Do you take anticonvulsant drugs (such as phenytoin, phenobarbital, or carbamazepine)?* These medications interfere with the activity of biotin in the body.

dermatitis, muscle pain, nausea, vomiting, hair loss, insomnia, and/or depression.

Toxicity

Toxicity has not been reported with biotin, even at doses as high as 10 mg per day.

Health Merits

Biotin has few substantiated uses as a treatment for medical conditions. High doses of this B vitamin have, however, been prescribed for babies who have a newborn form of seborrhea, an inflammation of the skin caused by oversecretion of oily substances.

How Much Biotin Do You Need?

Recommended Dietary Allowances have not been established for biotin.

Optimal Daily Allowance

Most research suggests that a dose of 30 to 100 mcg of biotin is safe and sufficient to meet the needs of all adults. We have concluded that anywhere within this range is acceptable as an ODA, but most people should aim to take 100 mcg per day.

Biotin Content of Common Foods

Food Item	*Amount of Vitamin (in mcg)*
Apple (1, raw)	1.66
Avocado (½, raw)	3.60
Banana (½, raw)	1.53

Food Sources

The best sources of biotin include liver, yeast, soy flour, egg yolks, fish, nuts, chocolate, and cheese.

Blackeye peas (⅓ cup)..3.86
Brazil nuts (1 oz) 3.12
Brie cheese (1 oz)..1.59
Broadbeans (⅓ cup, boiled) 1.19
Camembert cheese (1 oz)..2.15
Cashews (1 oz) 3.69
Chicken meat (3 oz, roasted) 1.70
Cod (3 oz, baked)..2.55
Egg (1 extra lg)..11.52
Grapefruit (½, raw)..1.20
Haddock (3 oz, steamed) 5.10
Halibut (3 oz, steamed)..4.25
Hazel nuts (1 oz) 21.55
Herring (3 oz, grilled) 8.51
Liver, beef (3 oz, fried) 45.08
Liver, chicken (3 oz, fried) 144.59
Macadamia nuts (1 oz)..1.70
Mackerel (3 oz, fried)..6.80
Mushrooms (½ cup, raw)..4.20
Oatmeal (½ cup)..24.57
Orange (1, raw) 1.31
Peanut butter (1 tbsp)...15.17
Peanuts (1 oz) 20.41
Pork chop (3 oz, grilled)...1.70
Salmon (3 oz, steamed) 3.40
Sardines, canned in oil (3 oz) 4.25
Sausage, beef (3 oz, fried) 1.70
Sausage, pork (3 oz, fried) 2.55
Strawberries (1 cup, fresh)...1.64
Tomato (½ cup, raw)..1.35
Tuna, canned in oil (3 oz)..2.55
Turkey, dark meat (3 oz, roasted) 1.70
Walnuts (1 oz)..5.39
Wheat germ (1 tbsp) 1.77
Yogurt, low-fat (1 cup) 6.58

How Much Biotin Are People in the United States Getting?

Few studies have been done on biotin consumption in the United States. According to one report on U.S. diets, however, biotin consumption ranges from 28 to 42 mcg per day.

How Much Biotin Are You Getting?

To determine whether you are reaching the ODA of riboflavin, use the information from the following list. For an explanation, refer back to "How Much Thiamin Are You Getting?" earlier in this chapter.

PERCENTAGE OF BIOTIN ODA

5 Percent

Haddock (3 oz, steamed)
Herring (3 oz, grilled)
Mackerel (3 oz, fried)
Walnuts (1 oz)
Yogurt, low-fat (1 cup)

10 Percent

Egg (1 extra lg)
Peanut butter (1 tbsp)

20 Percent

Hazelnuts (1 oz)
Oatmeal (½ cup)
Peanuts (1 oz)

40 Percent

Liver, beef (3 oz, fried)

100 Percent

Liver, chicken (3 oz, fried)

Our Recommendations

HOW MUCH BIOTIN DO YOU NEED TO ACHIEVE OPTIMAL HEALTH?

We advise consuming 30 to 100 mcg of biotin per day. Although anywhere within this range is acceptable, most people should aim for an optimal goal of 100 mcg per day.

WHAT SPECIAL CIRCUMSTANCES MIGHT AFFECT THE AMOUNT OF BIOTIN YOU NEED TO TAKE?

If you take anticonvulsant drugs, consume large amounts of raw egg whites, or are pregnant or breast-feeding, your target should be on the high end of our ODA range (100 mcg).

IS IT POSSIBLE TO CONSUME THE OPTIMAL AMOUNT OF BIOTIN THROUGH DIET ALONE?

One recent survey found that most people in the United States consume from 28 to 42 mcg of biotin per day. This is the low end of the ODA. To raise your intake, you can take biotin as part of many multivitamin preparations or in some B-complex tablets.

VITAMIN C

O ver the years, no other vitamin has received as much media attention, hype, and hoopla as vitamin C. Thanks in great part to its most prominent and outspoken advocate, Linus Pauling, millions of people religiously consume large amounts of vitamin C in hopes that it might cure them of everything from the common cold to cancer.

Despite all this attention, the average person isn't sure what to believe about this highly touted nutrient. Furthermore, until recently, most physicians weren't sure what to tell their patients. Research has now provided us with many of the answers.

Like the B vitamins, vitamin C is water-soluble, meaning that it dissolves in water. Excessive amounts are excreted in the urine.

Basic Functions

• Vitamin C is involved in the formation of connective tissue and bones. It also helps keep the body's tiny blood vessels (capillaries) strong and prevents them from bleeding.

• Vitamin C can promote the healing of wounds, particularly in the aftermath of surgery.

• Vitamin C stimulates the production of several important bodily hormones and brain chemicals.

• Vitamin C is an antioxidant and thus appears to help protect the body against some of the potentially damaging chemical reactions

History

The story of vitamin C is closely tied to scurvy, a potentially fatal disease with a history dating back to ancient times. During the height of the Roman Empire, soldiers involved in a two-year campaign along the Rhine River began experiencing sore and bleeding gums and loose teeth—symptoms that would later be identified with scurvy. The soldiers found a local plant, now believed to have been sorrel, which they began consuming in generous quantities and which cured the problem.

In subsequent centuries, identical symptoms resurfaced in the presence of poor nutrition. Most notably, crew members on long exploratory sea voyages during the 16th through 18th centuries were plagued with scurvy; their symptoms included soreness of the mouth and gums, weakness, and bleeding of the small blood vessels. In a journal entry in 1593, Sir Richard Hawkins described the deaths of 10,000 sailors from severe deficiencies associated with scurvy. In his desperate search for a treatment for this massive killer, Hawkins happened to administer oranges and lemons to his men and found that doing so reversed the condition. As effective as this treatment was, however, it fell out of favor for unknown reasons, and scurvy returned on a large scale, claiming many more lives over the next century.

Finally, in the mid-1700s, a physician named James Lind—who was surgeon of the British fleet—revived Hawkins' antidote to scurvy. Dr. Lind noted a low rate of scurvy on ships with food supplies that included citrus fruits, used primarily to flavor the large amounts of fish in the diet. Through experimentation, Dr. Lind clearly showed that scurvy-stricken sailors who ate two oranges and one lemon each day were ready to return to duty in about a week. He advised that lemon juice be added to the sailors' diets. When that occurred, the incidence of scurvy subsided dramatically. It has never completely disappeared, however; the condition is still present in emerging countries where nutritional deficiencies are commonplace.

Vitamin C was first isolated and identified in 1932 as the specific nutrient in fruits and vegetables responsible for preventing scurvy. At that time, it was called *ascorbic acid*.

of oxygen. In particular, it interferes with the production and activity of free radicals, toxic substances that seem to contribute to cell damage, disease, and aging. (See chapter 3, "Antioxidants.")

• Vitamin C plays a critical role in many aspects of the body's immune system. It stimulates the production of certain classes of antibodies, which are important for fighting illness and infection. It also promotes the production of natural compounds like interferon that can resist viral infections within the body.

• In high doses, vitamin C can minimize allergic reactions by interfering with the release of histamines. Vitamin C reduces the levels of histamine circulating in the blood.

• Vitamin C blocks the formation of nitrosamines, potentially cancer-causing compounds. Nitrosamines—produced in the stomach from chemicals (called nitrites) found in foods such as ham, sausages, and hot dogs—have been associated with an increased risk of certain cancers, especially those of the digestive system.

• Vitamin C is involved in the metabolism of folic acid. It is essential for converting the inactive form of folic acid into the active form.

• Vitamin C helps the body absorb iron by keeping the iron in an unoxidized form that is easier to use. If a person consumes vitamin C and iron at the same time, the body will better absorb the iron.

• Vitamin C influences the body's absorption of other minerals, too, sometimes increasing absorption and sometimes decreasing it. Vitamin C may slightly decrease the absorption of copper, for example. This may be particularly useful for people with the life-threatening condition called Wilson's disease, in which the body cannot rid itself of copper and thus is exposed to toxic levels of the mineral.

• Vitamin C stimulates the excretion of lead, thereby decreasing the concentration of lead in body tissues. High lead levels in the blood can cause serious problems, especially in children, including impaired intelligence.

Signs of Deficiency

Because the body cannot store vitamin C, you need to consume this potentially powerful nutrient regularly. Vitamin C is so plentiful in readily accessible fruits and vegetables, however, that serious deficiencies are rare in the United States and other developed countries. When a deficit does occur, symptoms do not develop overnight. In fact, they may not surface until shortages have persisted for several months—usually four to six.

Mild vitamin C deficits are more common than serious ones but are still relatively rare. Often they are associated with some illness or lifestyle habit that interferes with the body's intake or utilization of vitamin C. Smoking, stress, diabetes, and chronic diseases can increase the body's need for vitamin C. A mild deficiency may produce signs and symptoms such as fatigue, loss of appetite, muscle weakness, and susceptibility to infections.

Scurvy is the best-known disorder associated with severe deficits of vitamin C. The term *scurvy* comes from the Italian word *scorbutico*, which refers to an irritable, whining, discontented, neurotic person. When scurvy occurs (rarely in the United States), its symptoms include lethargy; fatigue; a change in personality; rough, dry, scaly skin; swollen, bleeding gums and lost teeth; hemorrhages of blood vessels; anemia (due to scurvy-related bleeding or poor iron absorption); slow healing of wounds; pain in the bones and joints; and increased susceptibility to infections.

Toxicity

In general, vitamin C appears to be relatively safe for most people, even when consumed in fairly large quantities over long periods of time. Doses as high as 10 g per day (more than 100 times the RDA) for several years do not have any toxic effect for some people. The body tends to excrete (in the urine) any vitamin C it can't put to use, thereby preventing toxic buildup. Some studies, however, have shown that toxic symptoms can occur in daily doses of as little as 1 g.

The most common symptom of excessive vitamin C consumption is gastrointestinal distress. Vitamin C can produce everything from an upset stomach to diarrhea (often accompanied by nausea and headaches). While this would concern most people, some vitamin C fanatics contend that the ideal dose of this nutrient is just

Who's at Risk for Vitamin C Deficiency?

If you answer yes to any of the following questions, you have an above-average risk of developing a vitamin C deficiency.

• *Do you smoke?* Studies show that smokers need at least twice as much vitamin C as nonsmokers, because smoking increases the rate of breakdown of this vitamin.

• *Are you an older person?* Older people often take medications that enhance the breakdown of vitamin C. In addition, many older people have poor dietary habits—sometimes because they are on limited budgets or because they live alone and do not cook much for themselves—and this compounds the problem. Finally, more vitamin C is required to fully saturate certain tissues (particularly white blood cells) in older people.

• *Do you have diabetes?* Studies show that diabetics have lower blood levels of vitamin C than nondiabetics. This is because ascorbic acid enters cells via the same protein carrier as glucose. When glucose levels are high, as in individuals with diabetes, glucose rather than ascorbic acid is transported, and ascorbic acid is excreted into the urine at a higher rate.

• *Do you drink a lot of alcohol?* Excessive alcohol consumption may cause vitamin C deficits for many reasons. Some researchers believe that alcohol itself destroys the vitamin, while others believe that another, undefined mechanism may be at work. Few argue about alcohol's effect upon overall nutrition; heavy users tend to replace nutritious, vitamin C–rich foods with alcohol.

below the diarrhea threshold. "You're not taking enough until you've started to get the runs," they claim. You can avoid diarrhea (and some other toxic symptoms) by increasing your vitamin C intake gradually—adding an extra 100 mg to your daily dose each week.

• *Are you pregnant or breast-feeding?* When the placenta transports vitamin C to the fetus during pregnancy, the mother's concentration of the vitamin tends to fall. When breast-feeding, a woman loses an average of 18 to 22 mg of vitamin C per day. She should increase her intake accordingly.

• *Are you a chronic user of certain medications?* Aspirin appears to interfere with the body's absorption of vitamin C. Although the effects of birth-control pills upon vitamin C are not understood, they may increase excretion of the vitamin in the urine. Other drugs, including tetracycline, increase the breakdown of vitamin C.

• *Are you exposed to high levels of environmental pollutants?* When pollutants are present, vitamin C is particularly important as an antioxidant. The vitamin is necessary for several enzyme systems that help detoxify pollutants (and drugs) and thus minimize their damaging effects. For this reason, you may need extra vitamin C under such circumstances.

• *Have you recently had surgery?* Immediately after an operation, the stress of surgery may produce physiological changes that lower vitamin C levels in the body.

• *Do you have an infectious disease?* Some infections create physiological changes that result in low levels of vitamin C in the bloodstream.

• *Are you on a faddish, imbalanced diet?* Many weight-loss programs are low in vitamin C.

• *Is your baby drinking a formula diet prepared at home with cow's milk?* Cow milk contains lower amounts of vitamin C than human milk. Your baby may require supplemental vitamin C if this is his or her diet.

Large doses of vitamin C might also increase your chances of developing kidney stones, in part by increasing the acidity of your urine, making it more conducive to the production of stones.

Large amounts of vitamin C in your system could interfere with tests that your doctor may conduct. You may get an erroneous result on a urine glucose test (used to screen for diabetes), for example, because of the large amounts of vitamin C excreted in your urine. The same "false negative" finding might occur on a fecal occult blood test (used to diagnose colon cancer).

Doctors have also reported a condition they call "rebound scurvy." This occurs in people who have consumed high doses of vitamin C and suddenly stop taking the supplement; when this happens, the body reacts as though it were continuing to receive large levels of the vitamin, breaking down and clearing the nutrient so rapidly that some symptoms of scurvy may surface.

Health Merits

Over the years, you've probably heard the claims that vitamin C is almost magical in its ability to fight both mild and serious diseases. A considerable body of research has been compiled on vitamin C—a much more credible source than the anecdotal reports relating to the vitamin. Some of the scientific research is persuasive and promising.

Inevitably, some of the claims for vitamin C have not panned out—at least not to the extent that its proponents would have you believe. But research does show that the vitamin can promote bone strength, help wounds heal, promote healthy gums, and reduce iron deficiency anemia (by enhancing absorption of iron). The vitamin may also protect against development of cataracts, cardiovascular disease, and some forms of cancer.

THE COMMON COLD

Despite years of pronouncements by respected scientists such as Linus Pauling, no clear-cut evidence exists that large doses of vitamin C can prevent or cure sneezes and sniffles. As far back as the 1970s, three well-conducted studies in Canada looked at the role of vitamin C in battling the common cold. Researchers found no positive effect on reducing the number of colds, though there was some evidence that people may miss fewer days at work if they take vitamin C to combat their upper respiratory infections. In other words, vitamin C doesn't seem to prevent colds, but it might help individuals recover more quickly. Large doses of the vitamin may also provide modest symptomatic relief, probably through an antihistamine effect.

CANCER

You don't have to look far to find support for consuming vitamin C to prevent cancer. As a recent editorial in a respected medical journal pointed out, large-scale studies have linked increased intake of vitamin C with a reduced risk of contracting several types of cancers.

Why does vitamin C seem to pack such a powerful punch against cancer? Researchers believe that vitamin C might have several anticancer mechanisms. Not only is it an antioxidant, thus able to deactivate free radicals, but also it improves the function of the immune system and prevents the formation of cancer-causing nitrosamines.

CANCER OF THE CERVIX

• Researchers at the Fred Hutchinson Cancer Research Center and the University of Washington, Seattle, calculated patient intake of vitamin C, as well as of vitamins A and E and folic acid, based on questionnaire responses by 189 women who had been diagnosed with cervical cancer and 227 cancer-free women. The data, published in 1989, indicate that high intakes of vitamin C were linked with a reduced risk of cervical cancer. Women who ranked in the highest 25 percent for vitamin C consumption were only half as likely to develop cervical cancer as women in the lowest 25 percent.

LUNG CANCER

• In a Finnish study published in 1991, researchers followed more than 4,500 men for 20 years to determine how their consumption of antioxidants influenced their risk of developing lung cancer. Over the two decades, 117 cases of lung cancer were diagnosed. Among nonsmoking men, those who consumed the least amount of vitamin C were three times more likely to develop lung cancer than those who consumed the most.

BREAST CANCER

• In a 1990 study, investigators at the University of Toronto and other major medical centers accumulated and analyzed data from a number of existing studies. Researchers hoped to sort out the conflicting conclusions of some of these other studies. The 1990 study showed that consuming large amounts of vitamin C substantially protected women against breast cancer. Women with the highest intakes were 31 percent less likely to develop breast cancer than women with the lowest intakes.

ORAL CANCER

• A 1988 study conducted at several U.S. research centers looked at the influence of vitamin C on 871 men and women with oral cancer and 979 cancer-free individuals. Diets rich in vitamin C were found to significantly protect individuals against cancer. Individuals who consumed the most vitamin C had a 40 to 50 percent lower risk than those who consumed the least.

OTHER FORMS OF CANCER

Gladys Block, a researcher at the University of California, Berkeley, School of Public Health, recently evaluated the wealth of scientific literature now available regarding the effect of vitamin C on cancer development. A few of her conclusions follow:

• All studies that have looked at the link between vitamin C and rectal cancer have concluded that higher intakes of this nutrient reduced the risk of cancer.

• Nine of 10 studies have found approximately a twofold decline in the likelihood of contracting cancers of the esophagus when vitamin C intake increased.

• Eight of nine studies concluded that increasing vitamin C intake leads to a decreased risk of stomach cancer.

• Positive results were also cited relative to vitamin C and prevention of cancers of the cervix, colon, lung, and pancreas. Vitamin C intake did not seem to significantly affect development of ovarian or prostate cancer, however.

CARDIOVASCULAR DISEASE

Vitamin C has shown a capacity to protect against cardiovascular disease in several ways. It has demonstrated an effect of lowering blood pressure. Some research has shown that it may also lower total cholesterol, raising HDL ("good") cholesterol and reducing LDL ("bad") cholesterol. A daily intake of 1 to 2 g of vitamin C has significantly increased HDL cholesterol levels.

CARDIOVASCULAR MORTALITY

• Using data from the First National Health and Nutrition Examination Survey (NHANES I) conducted by the National Center for Health Statistics between 1971 and 1975, scientists examined the relationship between vitamin C consumption and deaths caused by cardiovascular disease. Mortality attributed to cardiovascular disease was 42 percent less in men with the highest intake of vitamin C than in men with the lowest intake. In women, the difference was 25 percent. High intake of vitamin C reduced the number of deaths from all causes by 35 percent in men and 10 percent in women.

BLOOD PRESSURE

• In a 1984 study published by researchers in Japan, 194 men were divided into three groups based on their intake of vitamin C. The average systolic blood pressure reading of the men who consumed the most vitamin C was 7 percent lower than that of the men who consumed the least; the diastolic reading was 6 percent lower. Hypertension was seven times more common in the group taking the least amount of vitamin C than in the group taking the most.

• A 1988 Finnish study divided 722 men into four groups according to the levels of vitamin C in their blood. The mean systolic and diastolic blood pressure readings of the group with the highest vitamin C measurements were about 5 percent below those of the group with the lowest measurements.

CATARACTS

Eye fluids normally contain large amounts of vitamin C, but with aging, these levels decline. As that happens, proteins in the lens oxidize, making the lens more susceptible to clouding and the development of cataracts. But vitamin C may be able to protect against cataracts, or at least delay their onset.

• A 1991 study at Brigham and Women's Hospital, Boston, looked at the effects of vitamin C consumption on 77 men and women suffering from cataracts and on 35 cataract-free individuals. Low vitamin C intake was associated with an increased risk of developing cataracts. Individuals with intakes in the bottom 20 percent were four times more likely to develop cataracts than those in the top 20 percent. Blood levels of vitamin C showed a similar relationship: high blood levels seemed to provide significant protection against cataracts.

LONGEVITY

So far, no one is claiming that vitamin C is the elixir to produce a longer life. But if the evidence already cited here hasn't convinced you of the potential benefits of vitamin C, pay attention to the results of a study conducted by researchers at the University of California, Los Angeles, and published in 1992. These investigators examined the dietary habits—including intake of vitamin C from both foods and supplements—of more than 11,000 people, and then followed them for 10 years. The researchers concluded that men who consumed the most vitamin C (about 150 mg per day) had a 35 percent lower death rate over the next 10 years than men who consumed the least (about 30 mg per day). Women with the highest consumption had an overall death rate 10 percent lower than women with the lowest consumption. Data analysis showed that large amounts of vitamin C increased the life expectancy of men by six years and of women by one year.

How Much Vitamin C Do You Need?

When determining how much vitamin C you should take, keep in mind that environmental stress increases your need for this nutrient. So does the use of drugs, birth-control pills, and cigarettes. Also note that the most efficient way to attain maximum absorption, therefore, is to take vitamin C in multiple small doses.

Recommended Dietary Allowances

Infants

   0–6 months ....30 mg

   6–12 months ....35 mg

Children

   1–3 years ....40 mg

   4–10 years ....45 mg

Male and Female Adolescents and Adults

   11–14 years ....50 mg

   15+ years...60 mg

Pregnant Women

   ....70 mg

Lactating Women

   first 6 months ....95 mg

   second 6 months..90 mg

Optimal Daily Allowance

Although the RDA of vitamin C is only 60 mg for adults, we strongly believe that you can benefit from higher doses—perhaps about 10 times higher. We think that accumulating evidence that vitamin C protects against cardiovascular disease, some forms of cancer, and cataracts strengthens the case for taking higher doses of vitamin C.

We generally recommend an optimal range of 250 to 1,000 mg of vitamin C per day. For the average individual, we suggest a dose of 500 mg. If you are in one or more of the risk groups described in "Who's at Risk for Vitamin C Deficiency?" however, we advise you to move toward the high end of our range.

Vitamin C Content of Common Foods

Food Item	Amount of Vitamin (in mg)
Acerola (½ cup)	822
Acorn squash (1 cup, baked)	26
Broccoli (½ cup, boiled)	49
Brussels sprouts (4)	48
Butternut squash (1 cup, baked)	37

Food Sources

Vitamin C is widely available in both plant and animal foods. Fruits and vegetables such as green peppers, broccoli, potatoes, leafy green vegetables (spinach and turnips), strawberries, tomatoes, melons, oranges, and other citrus fruits are good sources of vitamin C. More modest levels of the nutrient are found in meat, poultry, fish, and dairy products. Grains do not contain vitamin C.

Note that the vitamin C content of any particular food item can vary, depending on factors such as growing conditions, time in storage, and cooking methods used. Vitamin C is highly unstable in the presence of heat, light, and water. Even chopping food into smaller sections can cause the loss of some vitamin C.

Cantaloupe (½ cup)..34
Cauliflower (½ cup, boiled)..34
Cranberry juice cocktail (8 oz) 108
Grapefruit (½ med) 47
Green peas (½ cup, raw) 31
Guava (1 med) 165
Honeydew melon (½ cup) 46
Kale (½ cup, boiled)..27
Kiwi fruit (1 med) 75
Lemon (1 med, raw) 31
Mango (1 med) 57
Marinara sauce (1 cup)..32
Orange (1 med)..80
Papaya (½ med)...94
Orange juice, from concentrate (8 oz) 97
Pineapple juice, canned (8 oz)...27
Potato (1 med, baked, with skin) 26
Potato (1 med, without skin)...20
Strawberries (½ cup)...43
Sweet pepper (½ cup, raw) 64
Grapefruit juice, canned (8 oz)...72
Sweet potato (1 med, baked)...28
Tangerine (1 med) 26
Tomato (1 med) 22
Tomato juice, canned (6 oz) 33

How Much Vitamin C Are People in the United States Getting?

In general, people in the United States consume much more than the RDAs of vitamin C. According to 1985 statistics, per capita intake of vitamin C was 114 mg, with more than 90 percent of it coming from fruits and vegetables. That was an increase from the 98 mg recorded in 1967–1969, probably because of the increased availability of citrus fruits and dark green vegetables and because of the fortification of certain foods. Some government statistics from the U.S. Department of Health and Human Services show that women ages 19 to 50 years consumed 187 percent of the RDA, compared to 207 percent for men.

In the Second National Health and Nutrition Examination Survey (NHANES II), with data published in the 1980s, researchers measured vitamin C in the blood. They found relatively few cases of low levels in children, and fewer deficiencies in women than in men. Overall, only 3 percent of people ages 3 to 74 years had low amounts of vitamin C in their blood.

How Much Vitamin C Are You Getting?

Before you decide that you need to take vitamin supplements or change the way you eat, you should know where you stand and how much improvement you really need. To help you analyze your current diet, we've developed a system you can use to calculate your approximate vitamin C intake. (You'll find this system in the other vitamin and mineral chapters, too.) Following is a list of vitamin C food sources, arranged according to the percentage of our Optimal Daily Allowance of vitamin C contained in them. Our ODA ranges from 250 to 1,000 mg; this self-test has been devised for an ODA of 500 mg, which works for most people. Since half a cup of broccoli contains 49 mg of vitamin C and the ODA for vitamin C is 500 mg, we've listed broccoli in the 10 Percent category. (We have erred on the conservative side when rounding off percentages.)

To determine your average daily intake of vitamin C, start by keeping an accurate food diary for three or four days. The longer you keep the diary, the more accurate your calculations will be. Write down exactly what you eat and drink, together with an estimate of the serving size. Don't concern yourself with precisely how much vitamin C each food item contains; simply use the list to find the food item and the percentage of the ODA that it provides. Then add up all these percentages to see if you reach 100 percent each day.

If a particular item in your meals is missing from this list (it would be impossible to include every food item here), use the nutritional information on the food packaging. Most packaged foods are required to list their vitamin contents on the label.

Remember that we have used 500 mg as the ODA in putting together this chart. If you have decided that your optimal dose falls elsewhere in our recommended range (from 250 to 1,000 mg), take that into account when calculating percentages. For example, based on the chart, a medium orange contains 10 percent of the vitamin C you need to reach a 500 mg ODA. But if your optimal dose is 1,000 mg, that orange meets only 5 percent of your RDA. If your ODA is 250 mg, the orange is in the 20 Percent category for you.

After you've determined how much vitamin C you are obtaining from your diet each day, you can calculate whether you need to take supplements to reach the ODA. Let's say that you determine that you are getting 30 percent of your vitamin C target through diet alone. You are consuming 150 mg of vitamin C in your diet (30 percent x 500 mg = 150 mg). To make up the difference, we would advise you to supplement your diet with 350 mg of vitamin C in tablet form (500 mg – 150 mg = 350 mg).

Because vitamin C is commonly sold in doses of 250, 500, and 1,000 mg, you may have difficulty getting supplements of the precise amount you want. We recommend that you come as close to your target as possible without taking several tablets to make things come out even. If you need a 350 mg supplement, you can go a little higher and take a 500 mg tablet, which will more than meet your needs without any real risk.

PERCENTAGE OF VITAMIN C ODA
(Based on 500 mg)
5 Percent

Acorn squash (1 cup, baked)
Brussels sprouts (4)
Butternut squash (1 cup, baked)

Cantaloupe (½ cup)
Cauliflower (½ cup, raw)
Grapefruit (½ med)
Green peas (½ cup, boiled)
Honeydew melon (½ cup)
Kale (½ cup, boiled)
Lemon (1 med, raw)
Marinara sauce (1 cup)
Pineapple juice, canned (8 oz)
Potato (1 med, baked, with skin)
Strawberries (½ cup)
Sweet potato (1 med, baked)
Tomato juice, canned (6 oz)

10 Percent

Breakfast cereals, most (²/₃ cup)
Broccoli (½ cup, boiled)
Grapefruit juice, canned (8 oz)
Kiwi fruit (1 med)
Mango (1 med)
Orange (1 med)
Papaya (½ med)
Product 19 (¾ cup)
Sweet pepper (½ cup, raw)
Total cereal (1 cup)

20 Percent

Cranberry juice cocktail (8 oz)
Orange juice, from concentrate (8 oz)

30 Percent

Guava (1 med)

100 Percent or More

Acerola (½ cup)

Our Recommendations

HOW MUCH VITAMIN C DO YOU NEED TO ACHIEVE OPTIMAL HEALTH?

We advise that you consume 250 to 1,000 mg of vitamin C per day. A daily intake of 500 mg will meet the optimal needs of most people.

WHAT SPECIAL CIRCUMSTANCES MIGHT AFFECT THE AMOUNT OF VITAMIN C YOU NEED TO TAKE?

If you have poor dietary habits, take multiple medications, have diabetes or an infectious disease, are recovering from surgery, smoke, are exposed to environmental pollutants, or are pregnant or breast-feeding, you should move toward the high end of our recommended intake of 250 to 1,000 mg per day.

IS IT POSSIBLE TO CONSUME THE OPTIMAL AMOUNT OF VITAMIN C THROUGH DIET ALONE?

To consume 500 mg of vitamin C per day through diet alone, you would have to drink five 8 ounce glasses of orange juice or ten 8 ounce glasses of grapefruit juice, for example. Most people find that it is more practical to obtain part of their vitamin C requirements through supplements.

VITAMIN D

Vitamin D is not like other vitamins. Because the body can manufacture this nutrient, in fact, vitamin D fails to meet the classic definition of a vitamin. Vitamin D is manufactured in the skin, with ultraviolet light driving the process. With regular exposure to sunlight, most people can manufacture enough of this vitamin to meet all of their needs. People who do not get enough year-round exposure, however, may require dietary D as well. Certain groups, including older people, have difficulty producing vitamin D themselves and may also require dietary D.

While rickets, a disease caused by a vitamin D deficiency, has been around for thousands of years, our knowledge of the vitamin itself has a relatively short history. It was first isolated and synthesized in the 1930s.

Forms of Vitamin D

The umbrella term *vitamin D* actually refers to a family of fat-soluble compounds. D vitamins, also called *calciferols*, come in many forms. Only two are important to the human body, however. These two—D_3 (a natural form) and D_2 (a synthetic form)—are equally useful to humans.

• Vitamin D_3, also called *cholecalciferol*, is formed when sunlight strikes the skin. This is the type of vitamin D contained in foods of animal origin.

• Vitamin D_2, or *ergocalciferol*, is produced through irradiation of a substance in plants called *ergosterol*. Vitamin D_2 is common in vitamin supplements and in fortified foods such as milk.

Basic Functions

• Vitamin D ensures that the body has enough calcium and phosphorous by increasing absorption of these minerals, both necessary for proper formation of bones and teeth; vitamin D also regulates the amounts of calcium and phosphorous in the blood.

• Vitamin D stimulates the production of insulin in the pancreas. People who have vitamin D deficiencies may not manufacture enough insulin to handle simple sugars (glucose), which may contribute to the development of diabetes.

• Vitamin D appears to be involved in the growth of cells essential to the body's immune system.

Signs of Deficiency

Vitamin D deficiencies are relatively common. Rickets, primarily a childhood disease, is the most widely acknowledged disorder associated with this type of deficiency. A similar condition in adults, called *osteomalacia*, involves the same kind of softening of the bones; it is produced by inadequate calcification—that is, by a lack of sufficient calcium in the bones.

Children with rickets often lose their appetite and grow slowly. Their muscles may be weak, and their weight-bearing bones may buckle, resulting in bowed legs and spinal deformities. Swollen joints, bone pain and tenderness, and delayed tooth eruption may also occur, as well as a greater susceptibility to tooth decay. Adults with osteomalacia may have some of the same symptoms, as well as bone fractures.

Toxicity

Can your body manufacture too much vitamin D if you spend a lot of time in the sun? The simple answer is no. While overexposure to the sun will dramatically raise your risk of developing skin cancer, it won't make you susceptible to toxic amounts of vitamin D. When your body has produced enough of that vitamin, a feedback system will automatically cut back the manufacturing process.

What about vitamin D supplements? Too much vitamin D taken this way *can* be toxic. This is because vitamin D is fat-soluble, so your body will retain excessive amounts rather than excrete them. Excessive amounts can persist in the body for weeks and even months.

In infants, doses as low as 1,800 IU per day can be toxic. In adults, symptoms of toxicity generally don't appear until much higher intake levels are reached—about 50,000 IU per day. Because young children can overdose at much lower levels than adults, be cautious about giving supplements to youngsters. Before giving your child vitamin D supplements, check with your pediatrician or family doctor. Some doctors do advise giving a supplement of up to 400 IU of vitamin D per day to breast-fed babies or babies

When There's Too Little Sun

Because the skin can manufacture vitamin D when it is exposed to sunlight, you may not require any vitamin D in your diet. Don't ignore dietary vitamin D completely, however, without thinking about your particular situation. How much time do you spend in the sun? How much of your skin is actually exposed to the sun? Do any environmental conditions—smog, fog, sunscreen, or window glass—keep ultraviolet light from reaching your skin? These are important factors in determining whether your body can produce all the vitamin D it needs.

If you're an older person, your skin produces vitamin D at about half the rate of the skin of a younger person. Skin pigment is important, too: to produce the same amount of vitamin D, people with dark skin require more sun exposure than people with light skin. The bodies of people living further from the equator also take longer to produce vitamin D.

Researchers use complicated formulas to calculate how fast your body manufactures vitamin D. These formulas need adjustment depending on the time of year and other factors, including those described here. In general, though, you need more than two hours of facial exposure per day in the winter months to meet your body's requirements, and less in the summer.

fed formula not fortified with vitamin D. Pediatricians also sometimes suggest supplements for older children—particularly those
who don't drink milk.

Who's at Risk for Vitamin D Deficiency?

If you answer yes to any of the following questions, you (or your
child) have an above-average risk of developing a vitamin D
deficiency.

• *Are you an older person?* Skin production of vitamin D tends to
slow down with age. Studies of older people—particularly older
women—show that as many as 75 percent are at marked risk for
vitamin D deficiencies.

• *Are you confined indoors and not exposed to sunlight?* With limited
sun exposure, your skin will produce a minimal amount of vitamin D, leaving you to rely on diet alone for your vitamin D needs.

• *Do you have kidney or liver disease?* Vitamin D, formed in the skin,
must be modified chemically in the kidney and liver before the
body can use it. This process can be severely impaired if these
organs are diseased.

• *Do you regularly take certain medications such as cholesterol-lowering drugs (cholestyramine or colestipol), mineral oil, or anticonvulsants
(phenytoin, phenobarbital, or primidone)?* Cholesterol-lowering
agents and mineral oil impair the body's ability to absorb vitamin D. Anticonvulsants cause conversion of the vitamin to an
inactive form.

• *Do you drink large amounts of alcohol?* Alcohol appears to reduce
blood levels of vitamin D and lower absorption by the intestines.

• *Do you drink fewer than three glasses of milk per day?* Except
through fortified dairy products such as milk, it is difficult to get
adequate quantities of vitamin D routinely in the diet.

• *Are you pregnant or breast-feeding?* According to the RDAs, pregnant or breast-feeding women need an extra 200 IU of vitamin D
per day.

• *Is your child being breast-fed and not being exposed regularly to the
sun?* According to the RDAs, breast-fed infants without regular sun
exposure should get a supplement of 200 IU of vitamin D per day.

Common signs of overdosing may be relatively mild, such as nausea, weakness, headaches, and constipation. A more serious complication is the formation of calcium deposits in the heart, blood vessels, and kidneys.

Health Merits

Vitamin D prevents and cures rickets. Researchers believe it is also good for cardiovascular health, because, for example, it may help to control high blood pressure. Some of the strongest evidence regarding benefits of this vitamin, however, relate to its ability to protect against osteoporosis (the thinning of bones) and fractures. By helping to maintain adequate levels of calcium in the bloodstream, vitamin D promotes bone mineralization, which strengthens bones. Together with calcium and estrogen, vitamin D helps to ensure healthy bones.

OSTEOPOROSIS

Because osteoporosis is so common, disabling, and even life threatening, most doctors urge older female patients to consume adequate amounts of vitamin D. Several studies have convinced physicians to make this recommendation.

• In a 1987 study conducted in Amsterdam, the Netherlands, researchers evaluated the role of vitamin D supplements in preventing hip fractures in both men and women. They studied the blood levels of vitamin D in 125 older men and women with hip fractures, and in 74 without fractures. Vitamin D levels were notably lower in individuals with hip fractures.

• In a 1991 study at Tufts University, Boston, Massachusetts, postmenopausal women received either 400 IU of vitamin D supplements per day or a placebo. Each woman also received 377 mg of calcium supplements per day. Researchers measured the bone density in these women every six months. After one year, the women treated with vitamin D had modest increases in their bone mineral density. The women who received the placebo showed no significant effects. The benefits were most noticeable during the last six months of the study—from December/January through June/July, when the body's own production of vitamin D tends to be lower because of decreased sun exposure.

Rickets: A Rare But Crippling Disease

Vitamin D has what is called antirachitic activity. *Antirachitic* is a fancy word meaning "having the ability to prevent or cure rickets," the childhood disease most closely associated with vitamin D deficiency.

Rickets is a bone disease that is probably nearly as old as the human species. The bones of people who have this condition soften and become so pliable that they bend, which can cause skeletal problems such as knock-knees, bowlegs, and pelvic and spine deformities. Rickets can also produce misshapen breastbones and "sunken" chests that can lead to serious lung and breathing difficulties.

Although vitamin D itself has only been known since the 1930s, the first scientific descriptions of rickets date back to the mid-1600s. Rickets became a serious problem during the industrial revolutions of northern Europe and England, in the early 1800s, when air pollution prevented sunshine from reaching people living in urban areas.

Rickets is more than just a vitamin D problem; it also involves calcium. The bodies of people who have rickets cannot absorb enough calcium, either because these people do not have enough calcium in their diets or because they do not have enough vitamin D to absorb the calcium.

Rickets is rare in most parts of the world today, thanks largely to the availability of foods rich in vitamin D, either naturally or through fortification. Children who are breast-fed for a long time without vitamin D supplementation do have an increased chance of developing this disease, however. Rickets occurs most commonly today in children under three years of age.

• In a 1992 study in Lyon, France, 3,270 elderly women received either (1) 800 IU of vitamin D and a 1.2 g supplement of calcium per day or (2) two placebo pills. After 18 months, the women who had received vitamin D and calcium had suffered 43 percent fewer hip fractures and 32 percent fewer other nonvertebral fractures (of the wrist, forearm, humerus, and pelvis) than those who had received placebos.

How Much Vitamin D Do You Need?

Recommended Daily Allowances for vitamin D are given here in both micrograms and international units. The IU is a common unit of measurement among many vitamin supplement manufacturers. Remember that people who get enough sunlight do not need additional vitamin D.

Optimal Daily Allowance

We recommend an optimal daily allowance of 400 IU of vitamin D per day. Fewer foods are rich in vitamin D than in other vitamins and minerals, so you may need to take a vitamin D tablet to supplement your diet.

Recommended Dietary Allowances

	mcg	IU
Infants		
0–6 months	5	300
Children		
6 months–10 years	10	400
Male and Female Adolescents and Adults		
11–24 years	10	400
25+ years	5	200
Pregnant Women		
	10	400
Lactating Women		
	10	400

Although the risks of toxicity may be low at moderately higher doses, we do not recommend supplemental intakes of more than 400 IU.

Vitamin D Content of Common Foods

Food Item	Amount of Vitamin (in IU)
Bran Flakes cereal (½ cup)	14.8
Brie cheese (1 oz)	2.4
Butter (1 tsp)	1.6
Camembert cheese (1 oz)	2.0
Cheddar cheese (1 oz)	2.8
Cod liver oil (1 tbsp)	1,145.6
Corn Flakes cereal (½ cup)	9.6
Cream cheese (1 oz)	3.2
Edam cheese (1 oz)	2.0
Egg (1)	36.4
Feta cheese (1 oz)	5.6
Gouda cheese (1 oz)	2.8

Food Sources

Although some foods naturally contain vitamin D—including eggs, butter, oily fish (salmon, herring, and sardines), liver, and cod liver oil—most dietary vitamin D comes from foods that have been fortified. Cow milk, for example, is usually fortified with vitamin D and is the primary source of dietary vitamin D for children. Infant formula is also fortified with vitamin D. (Breast milk contains little D.) Other commonly fortified foods include margarine and ready-to-eat breakfast cereals.

Plants are not good sources of vitamin D. Green leafy vegetables, for example, contain only small amounts of this vitamin.

Vitamin D is a remarkably stable nutrient; little of it is lost during cooking and storage.

Herring, grilled (3 oz) 850.4
Ice cream, vanilla (½ cup) 3.2
Mackerel, fried (3 oz) 718.0
Margarine (1 tsp)...14.8
Parmesan cheese (1 oz) 2.8
Sardines, canned (3 oz) 255.2
Special K cereal (½ cup) 12.0
Tuna, canned in oil (3 oz)...197.2

How Much Vitamin D Are People in the United States Getting?

Little information exists on vitamin D consumption; data that are available deal primarily with intake among children. Statistics in the most recent (1989) edition of *Recommended Dietary Allowances*, published by the National Research Council, indicate that individuals who drink three 8 ounce glasses of milk per day get about 7.5 mcg (300 IU) of vitamin D from that source, plus small amounts from other food sources and whatever their bodies produce if exposed to the sun. Children are the biggest milk drinkers in the population.

Because adults tend to drink less milk, the U.S. Department of Agriculture reports, they get much less vitamin D from fortified milk. Women average about 2.1 mcg and men about 1.5 mcg.

How Much Vitamin D Are You Getting?

Before you decide that you need to take vitamin supplements or change the way you eat, you should know where you stand and how much improvement you really need. To help you analyze your current diet, we've developed a system you can use to calculate your approximate vitamin D intake. (You'll find this system in the other vitamin and mineral chapters, too.) Following is a list of vitamin D food sources, arranged according to the percentage of our Optimal Daily Allowance of vitamin D contained in them. Since 3 ounces of tuna canned in oil contain 197.2 IU of vitamin D and the ODA for vitamin D is 400 IU, we've listed tuna in the 50 Percent category.

To determine your average intake of vitamin D, start by keeping an accurate food diary for three or four days. The longer you keep the diary, the more accurate your calculations will be. Write down exactly what you eat and drink, together with an estimate of the serving size. Don't concern yourself with precisely how much vitamin D each food item contains; simply use the list to find the food item and the percentage of the ODA that it provides. Then add up all these percentages to see if you reach 100 percent each day.

If a particular item in your meals is missing from this list (it would be impossible for us to include every food item here), use the nutritional information on the food packaging. Most packaged foods are required to list their vitamin contents on the label.

After you've determined how much vitamin D you are obtaining from your diet each day, you can calculate whether you need to take supplements to reach the ODA. Let's say that you determine that you are getting 60 percent of your vitamin D target through diet alone. You are consuming 240 IU of vitamin D in your diet (60 percent x 400 IU = 240 IU). To make up the difference, we would advise you to supplement your diet with 160 IU of vitamin D in tablet form (400 IU – 240 IU = 160 IU).

Because vitamin D is commonly sold in doses of 100, 200, or 400 IU, you may have difficulty finding a supplement in the precise amount you want. We recommend that you get as close as you can to your supplemental needs without taking several pills and/or cutting them in half. In the example cited here, you can meet your 160 IU requirements by taking a 200 IU tablet of vitamin D, which will more than meet your needs without any real risk (in this case, don't be concerned about going a little higher than your optimal intake).

PERCENTAGE OF VITAMIN D ODA

10 Percent

Egg (1)

50 Percent

Tuna, canned in oil (3 oz)

60 Percent

Sardines, canned (3 oz)

100 Percent or More

Mackerel (3 oz, fried)
Herring (3 oz, grilled)
Cod liver oil (1 tbsp)

Our Recommendations

HOW MUCH VITAMIN D DO YOU NEED TO ACHIEVE OPTIMAL HEALTH?

We recommend that you consume 400 IU of vitamin D each day.

WHAT SPECIAL CIRCUMSTANCES MIGHT AFFECT THE AMOUNT OF VITAMIN D YOU NEED TO TAKE?

If you are an older person, are confined indoors, have kidney or liver disease, do not drink milk, take certain cholesterol-lowering or anticonvulsant medications, drink large amounts of alcohol, or are pregnant or breast-feeding, you may need to be particularly conscientious about consuming your optimal dose of vitamin D.

IS IT POSSIBLE TO CONSUME THE OPTIMAL AMOUNT OF VITAMIN D THROUGH DIET ALONE?

It is possible to consume 400 IU of vitamin D per day, but many people do not do so, partly because there are few vitamin D–rich foods. Most people find that they need to supplement their dietary intake with a vitamin D capsule each day, no matter how much sun exposure they feel they get.

VITAMIN E

Vitamin E has grabbed its share of headlines in recent years. In fact, few nutrients have been the subject of as much discussion as this one. According to the most zealous vitamin proponents, vitamin E is nothing short of a magic pill capable of everything from enhancing one's sex life to stopping the aging process in its tracks.

You shouldn't be surprised to learn that many of these claims have little if any scientific support behind them. Still, a growing body of evidence shows that vitamin E does have significant health benefits. This chapter will help you sort scientific fact from fiction regarding this much-discussed vitamin.

Basic Functions

• Vitamin E can neutralize the free radicals that are released constantly as the body utilizes oxygen, especially during times of physical stress. Without this type of intervention, these free radi-

Forms of Vitamin E

Vitamin E is actually a generic term for several fat-soluble compounds, collectively called *tocopherols* and *tocotrienols*. The term for the most common and active of the tocopherols, *alpha-tocopherol*, is often used interchangeably with *vitamin E*. The other tocopherols (such as beta-, delta-, and gamma-tocopherol) differ slightly in chemical structure and generally have lower vitamin E activity.

cals would damage cells and increase the probability that certain diseases or degenerative processes (such as cancer, cataracts, atherosclerosis, and aging) would occur.

• In its role as an antioxidant, vitamin E protects the lungs against injury from air pollution. It also preserves tissues throughout the body and may impede the development of tumors. Because cell membranes throughout the body are made up of fatty acids—which are highly susceptible to oxidative attack—the antioxidative properties of vitamin E can keep these cells from being damaged. (Since vitamin E is fat-soluble, it functions most effectively in an environment like the cell membranes.)

• Vitamin E works as an ally of vitamin A, vitamin C, and carotene, preventing their destruction through oxidation. Vitamin E itself appears to function more effectively if other antioxidants (such as vitamin C) are present.

History

In 1922, researchers stumbled upon a mysterious substance in lettuce and wheat germ that played an important role in the reproduction of rats. The scientists had been observing female rats that had been placed on a restricted diet consisting of rancid lard; while these rats were able to ovulate and conceive, their fetuses typically died. Once lettuce or wheat germ was added to the diet, however, normal reproduction occurred. The scientists could not identify the specific chemical substance in these foods but named it "Factor X."

Efforts to identify Factor X continued for several years. Meanwhile, additional animal studies showed that male rats also developed reproductive abnormalities, including atrophy of the testicles, when fed a diet deficient in this substance. For a time, this elusive nutrient was called the "antisterility vitamin." Finally, in 1936, vitamin E was isolated and named.

Signs of Deficiency

Serious vitamin E deficiencies tend to be rare in the United States. Not only is vitamin E common in most diets, but the body's tissues store reserves of this nutrient. You must consume low levels of vitamin E for literally months to years, therefore, before signs of a deficiency occur.

When a vitamin E deficiency does occur, often in conjunction with inflammatory bowel disease, it can impair a number of bodily functions, including those involved with the reproductive system, nervous system, and muscle tissues. Some of the most common signs are loss of appetite; difficulty walking (which occurs when free radicals damage the cerebellum and brain stem, partly because antioxidants, such as vitamin E, are too scarce to protect the nerves); anemia (in which the life span of red blood cells is shortened because red blood cell membranes are susceptible to oxidative attack); mild gastrointestinal distress, such as nausea; eye problems, including cataracts and retinal problems; and impairment of the reproductive system, including testicular deterioration, fertility loss, and increased chance of fetal death (spontaneous abortion).

Toxicity

When it comes to vitamin E, you don't need to worry much about toxicity. Even in doses far above those recommended by the government, few problems have been associated with taking this vitamin. There are virtually no side effects of doses up to 800 IU. In many trials, doses up to 3,200 mg (or about 5,000 IU) per day have produced relatively few adverse effects.

Adverse reactions have been reported at extremely high doses. They have included fatigue; nausea; headache; double vision; weak muscles; breast tenderness in women; intestinal cramps and diarrhea, and emotional disturbances such as depression, fatigue, and mood swings. At high doses vitamin E can also interfere with the potency of anticoagulants, medications prescribed most often to prevent blood clotting in patients with heart disease.

Who's at Risk for Vitamin E Deficiency

If you answer yes to any of the following questions, you (or your baby) have an above-average risk of developing a vitamin E deficiency.

• *Do you have any of the following chronic illnesses: cystic fibrosis, pancreatitis, biliary cirrhosis, or Crohn's disease?* These illnesses can produce vitamin E deficiencies, particularly when they interfere with absorption of fat from the intestines. In general, however, this poor absorption must persist for five to ten years before signs of a deficiency occur.

•*Is your diet high in polyunsaturated fatty acids (found in corn, safflower, and sunflower oil)?* Vitamin E protects these unsaturated fats from oxidation. When you consume more of them, you need extra vitamin E to maintain this protective role.

• *Are you on a weight-loss (e.g. low-fat, low-calorie) diet?* Inadequate amounts of vitamin E might be consumed while dieting.

• *Do you take certain medications that interfere with vitamin E absorption?* Most commonly, these deficits occur with mineral oil and particular anticholesterol drugs such as cholestyramine and colestipol, when they are taken for long periods of time.

• *Do you smoke cigarettes?* Smoking increases the likelihood of vitamin E insufficiency.

• *Are you exposed to air pollution?* Living in a community with high levels of smog and other environmental pollutants can increase the need for vitamin E.

• *Are you pregnant or breast-feeding?* Extra vitamin E is necessary to ensure proper fetal growth. The RDAs advise a 25 percent increase of this vitamin during pregnancy. Women who are nursing should increase the dose even more.

• *Was your baby born prematurely, with a low birth weight?* A preterm infant may have difficulty absorbing vitamin E and may also have low amounts of the vitamin stored in the liver.

Health Merits

Keeping up with all of the recent research into the potential health benefits of vitamin E is difficult. The impressive findings of the best of this research, however, are impossible to ignore.

CANCER

A growing body of research indicates that vitamin E can provide protection against a variety of cancers, including oral, lung, cervical, and breast cancers. For example, an eight-year Finnish study of 36,265 adults concluded that individuals with low blood levels of alpha-tocopherol (vitamin E) were 1.5 times more likely to develop cancer than people with higher amounts.

Skeptics point to vitamin E research that has not shown protective effects against cancer. Even some of these reports, however, have found that cancer-free people have higher blood levels of vitamin E than individuals with cancer, although the differences may not be great enough to have what researchers call "statistical significance."

Why might vitamin E play a role in preventing cancer? Several mechanisms may be at work, but vitamin E's role as an antioxidant is probably at the forefront. Vitamin E appears to be able to neutralize the potentially damaging free radicals formed in the body as part of the process in which cells use oxygen. In addition, this vitamin apparently blocks formation of cancer-promoting compounds (carcinogens) called nitrosamines, and it can stimulate the body's disease-battling immune system.

ORAL/THROAT CANCER

• In 1992, researchers at the National Cancer Institute compared the use of vitamin supplements by 1,114 patients with oral and pharyngeal (throat) cancer to the use by 1,268 cancer-free individuals. This study indicated that use of vitamin E supplements reduces an individual's chance of developing these cancers. People who used vitamin E supplements regularly for six or more months were only half as likely to develop these cancers as people who had never taken vitamin E pills regularly.

LUNG CANCER

• A study at Louisiana State University Medical Center, published in 1990, involved 59 people with newly diagnosed lung cancer. Their vitamin blood levels—including vitamin E—were compared with those of a similar number of cancer-free individuals. The lung cancer patients had significantly lower amounts of vitamin E in their blood.

• In a study in Washington County, Maryland, researchers at the Johns Hopkins School of Hygiene and Public Health drew and froze blood samples from more than 25,000 people. In the ensuing years, 99 of those people developed lung cancer. Levels of vitamin E in the blood samples of those with cancer were compared to levels in the blood samples of 196 cancer-free individuals, and the average vitamin E levels were significantly lower in those with cancer. Researchers, who published their data in 1991, concluded that subjects with vitamin E blood levels ranking in the lowest 20 percent had 2.5 times more risk of developing lung cancer than those whose levels were in the highest 20 percent.

• In Finland, scientists from many institutions followed 4,538 men for 20 years after performing initial screening and dietary exams. The goal was to determine whether the intake of antioxidant nutrients by these men influenced their chances of developing lung cancer. During this period, 117 cases of lung cancer were diagnosed. Among nonsmokers, according to findings published in 1991, those who consumed the lowest amounts of vitamin E were three times more likely to develop lung cancer than those who took the highest doses. Vitamin E did not seem to protect smokers against cancer.

• One other study deserves some attention here: a 1994 study, conducted in the United States and Finland, in which scientists looked at the effects of Vitamin E and beta-carotene upon long-term smokers. Through this widely publicized study, discussed in more detail in the vitamin A chapter, (see "Health Merits—Lung Cancer") researcher's reached the unexpected conclusion that neither vitamin E nor beta-carotene protected smokers from lung cancer. They did find, however, that fewer cases of prostate cancer occurred in men who took vitamin E.

CANCER OF THE CERVIX

• In the Seattle area of the state of Washington, 189 women diagnosed with cervical cancer and 227 cancer-free women filled out dietary questionnaires. They provided information about their intake of vitamins A, C, and E, folic acid, and other nutritional substances. In a study published in 1989, researchers linked consumption of large amounts of vitamin E with a reduced risk of cervical cancer. Women in the top 25 percent of vitamin E intake were only one-third as likely to have cancer as those in the bottom 25 percent.

• At the start of a 1991 study at the Albert Einstein College of Medicine in New York, researchers drew blood from 116 women: 36 had no cervical disease, and the other 80 had abnormal Pap smears, but their detected lesions had not yet progressed to cancer. In evaluations of the antioxidant levels in these blood samples, vitamin E measurements were found to be significantly lower in women with cervical dysplasia (irregular cells that may proceed to cancer) than in women with normal Pap smears. This relationship was graded; women having the most severe lesions (closest to cancer) had the lowest levels of vitamin E.

BREAST CANCER

• In a 1984 study at the Medical College of St. Bartholomew's Hospital in London, England, researchers drew blood samples from more than 5,000 women and then monitored the women for the development of breast cancer. Over the next several years, 39 of the women developed breast cancer. Their blood antioxidant levels were compared to the levels of 78 women who had remained free of cancer. Low levels of vitamin E were associated with a much higher risk of cancer. Women with the lowest vitamin E levels were five times more likely to have cancer than women with the highest levels.

We do not believe that any single study refutes all the positive research about vitamin E. Keep in mind that the dose of vitamin E in the U.S./Finnish study was far less than our optimal recommendation for this nutrient and less than the dose contained in most supplements. In addition, all participants in this study were cigarette smokers—suggesting that a person who continues negative health behaviors can't necessarily expect vitamins to overcome them.

CARDIOVASCULAR DISEASE

Several studies have shown that vitamin E may offer protection from heart disease. Researchers suspect that vitamin E helps protect against hardening of the arteries (atherosclerosis) by preventing the oxidation of LDL (low-density lipoprotein) cholesterol. This is the so-called bad cholesterol that causes the buildup of fatty deposits in the walls of the arteries.

Two major studies appear to support this thesis. Both were conducted by investigators at Harvard Medical School and the Harvard School of Public Health.

• In the Health Professionals Study, nearly 40,000 male health workers—ages 40 to 75 years and all free of heart disease—filled out dietary questionnaires in 1986 that asked for information about their intake of a variety of nutrients, including antioxidants such as vitamin E. Over the next four years, 667 cases of coronary disease (heart attacks or coronary arteries requiring angioplasty) were diagnosed among these men. After analyzing these cases, researchers concluded that men in the top fifth of vitamin E consumption had a 41 percent lower risk of coronary disease than men in the bottom fifth. According to the study, published in 1993, men who consumed 100 to 249 IU per day were best protected; men who took 100 IU or more of vitamin E supplements for at least two years had a 37 percent lower risk of heart disease than those who did not take supplements.

• The Nurses' Health Study looked at the effect of antioxidants on heart disease in women. In 1980, more than 87,000 female nurses—ages 34 to 59 years and all free of heart disease—filled out dietary questionnaires. Within eight years, 552 of these women were diagnosed with coronary heart disease. Data published in 1993 indicate that women with the highest intake of vitamin E (via supplementation) had 34 percent less chance of major heart disease than those with the lowest intake. The risk of coronary disease in women who had used vitamin E supplements for two or more years was 41 percent lower than in nonusers.

IMMUNITY

Your body's ability to knock out invading bacteria, viruses, and other disease-causing agents depends on the strength of your immune system. Studies show that vitamin E deficits can undermine the functioning of that disease-battling system and may increase your body's vulnerability to a variety of disorders, from infections in older people to cancers associated with increasing age. In fact, some research confirms that vitamin E supplements may improve the workings of the immune system.

• Thirty-two healthy men and women—ages 60 years and over—participated in a 1990 study at Tufts University in Boston to evaluate the effect of vitamin E on immunity. They were given either a placebo or 800 IU of vitamin E each day for a month. By the end of that period, several measures of immune function had improved in the group receiving vitamin E; subjects receiving only the placebo experienced no such changes.

CATARACTS

Cataracts, characterized by a clouding of the lens of the eye, are a leading cause of blindness among older people. Some research suggests that vitamin E, in conjunction with carotenoids and vitamin C, may effectively postpone the development of cataracts. These antioxidants seem to interfere with the oxidation of proteins in the lens and thus may block the processes that lead to clouding of the lens.

• In a 1991 study, researchers at the University of Western Ontario, Canada, examined the use of vitamin supplements in 175 people with cataracts and in 175 cataract-free individuals. The patients with cataracts were 44 percent less likely to have consumed vitamin E supplements than their counterparts without cataracts.

• In a 1992 study in Finland, researchers examined antioxidant blood levels of 47 men and women with cataracts and of 94 cataract-free men and women. Low amounts of vitamin E (and of beta-carotene) were associated with an increased risk of developing cataracts. Individuals having vitamin E levels in the lowest third had a 90 percent greater chance of having cataracts than those in the highest two-thirds.

PARKINSON'S DISEASE

Scientists have many theories about the cause of Parkinson's disease, a degenerative disorder involving the nerve centers of the brain. One of the most popular theories is that Parkinson's is a disease of self-destruction, in which nerve cells produce toxins (such as free radicals) that then damage and kill the cells themselves. If this is true, then doses of vitamin E—with its capacity as an antioxidant—may retard and halt the process.

•In a small study at Columbia University College of Physicians and Surgeons, New York, published in 1991, patients in the early stages of Parkinson's disease received large doses of vitamins E (3,200 mg a day) and C (3,000 mg a day). Doctors hoped that these nutrients might slow progression of the disease, and in fact, that's precisely what happened. Patients taking these antioxidants were able to remain medication free for extended periods of time; because their illness progressed more slowly, they were able to postpone starting treatment with a drug called levadopa for a full two-and-a-half years. However, a larger study using only vitamin E (2,000 I.U. a day) has failed to demonstrate that this nutrient slows the progression of Parkinson's disease.

How Much Vitamin E Do You Need?

Vitamin E requirements vary according to two factors: (1) the body size of the individual and (2) the amount of polyunsaturated fats the individual consumes. Vitamin E is necessary to protect polyun-

Recommended Dietary Allowances

	Alpha-TE * (in mg)	IU *
Infants		
0–6 months	3	5
6–12 months	4	6
Children		
1–3 years	6	9
4–10 years	7	11
Male Adolescents and Adults		
11+ years	10	15
Female Adolescents and Adults		
11+ years	8	12
Pregnant Women		
	10	15
Lactating Women		
first 6 months	12	18
second 6 months	11	17

Several different units of measurement have been used to quantitate amounts of vitamin E. The most common measures are alpha-TE (alpha-tocopherol equivalents) and IU (international units). Alpha-TE is expressed in milligrams (mg), per formal RDA guidelines. For your convenience, we have also listed approximate IU equivalents.

saturated fats in bodily tissues from oxidation. Thus, the more polyunsaturates in the diet, the greater the need for vitamin E.

Because of these individual differences, specific vitamin E recommendations for the population at large are difficult to make. The Recommended Dietary Allowances on the preceding page are general guidelines based on averages for healthy individuals.

Optimal Daily Allowance

Serious deficiencies of vitamin E are rare in the United States, so the primary consideration in choosing a dose of this vitamin is promotion of optimal health. Studies clearly show that doses far above the RDAs have beneficial health effects. High doses can reduce the risks of chronic disease and improve functioning of the immune system, among other things.

Food Sources

Vitamin E is available in both animal and plant products. As a rule, plant products contain more vitamin E than animal products do. In addition, meats from animals that have diets high in fat may also be good sources of vitamin E, but because of their high fat content, you're better off finding vitamin E in plants.

What are the best sources of vitamin E? Vegetable and seed oils (such as sunflower, soybean, and cottonseed) are all particularly rich in vitamin E, but the distribution of vitamin E compounds differs from one type of oil to another. While the vitamin E content of safflower oil is 90 percent alpha-tocopherol (the most biologically active of the vitamin E compounds), for example, corn oil has just 10 percent alpha-tocopherol. Other good sources of vitamin E are green leafy vegetables, liver, whole grains, wheat germ, butter, margarine, egg yolk, and nuts.

Remember that cooking can deplete vitamin E content. Cooking for long periods of time at high temperatures can destroy the vitamin E in oils.

We have selected 100 to 400 IU per day as a range for an Optimal Daily Allowance (ODA) of vitamin E. Although anything within this range is acceptable, 400 IU is safe and may be optimal if you have one or more of the deficiency risks listed in "Who's at Risk for Vitamin E Deficiency?" If your risks of deficiency are low, you might choose an ODA at the low end of our recommended scale.

Vitamin E Content of Common Foods

Food Item	*Amount of Vitamin (in IU)*
Acorn squash (1 cup, baked)	2.42
Almond oil (1 tbsp)	8.16
Almonds (¼ cup)	11.33
Apricots (3 med)	1.41
Asparagus (½ cup, raw)	2.00
Bagel (1 med)	2.70
Bass (3½ oz, baked/broiled)	1.50
Blue cheese dressing (1 tbsp)	1.65
Blueberries (½ cup, fresh)	2.04
Bluefish (3½ oz, baked/broiled)	1.50
Brown rice (1 cup)	2.10
Butternut squash (1 cup, baked)	2.42
California avocado (½)	2.49
Canola oil (1 tbsp)	13.47
Cashews (¼ cup)	3.86
Chocolate (1 oz)	2.52
Cod (3½ oz, baked/broiled)	1.95
Corn oil (1 tbsp)	21.21
Cottage cheese (1 cup)	2.18
Cottonseed oil (1 tbsp)	13.26
Dandelion greens (½ cup, cooked)	1.76
Filberts (¼ cup)	12.11
French dressing (1 tbsp)*	6.60
Garbanzo beans (½ cup, cooked)	2.46
Green peas (½ cup, cooked)	2.55
Hazelnuts (¼ cup)	12.11

Italian dressing (1 tbsp)*..6.60
Kale (½ cup, cooked) 4.02
Lima beans (½ cup, cooked)..2.03
Macadamia nuts (¼ cup) 8.25
Mackerel (3½ oz, baked/broiled) 2.28
Mango (1, fresh) 3.48
Margarine, regular (1 tbsp)...2.34
Margarine, spread (1 tbsp) 1.76
Mayonnaise (1 tbsp) 1.53
Milk, whole (8 oz) 11.55
Mustard greens (½ cup, cooked) 2.25
Navy beans (½ cup, cooked) 1.53
Oil and vinegar dressing (1 tbsp)*....................................4.50
Olives, black (10)...1.80
Oysters (1 cup, raw) 3.06
Palm oil (1 tbsp) 5.31
Peach (1 med) 1.35
Peanut butter (2 tbsp)...3.08
Peanut oil (1 tbsp)...3.75
Peanuts (¼ cup)...5.48
Pecans (¼ cup)..1.38
Perch (3½ oz, baked/broiled)...1.95
Pine nuts (1 oz)..2.55
Potato chips (about 14)..2.81
Prunes (10, dried)..3.15
Pumpkin, canned (½ cup)..1.65
Ranch dressing (1 tbsp)*...3.75
Russian dressing (¼ tbsp)* 5.70
Safflower oil (1 tbsp) 7.76
Salmon (3 oz, baked/broiled) 2.01
Sesame oil (1 tbsp) 5.91
Skim milk (8 oz) 11.25
Sole (3 oz, baked/broiled) 2.40
Soybean oil (1 tbsp) 21.21
Soybeans (½ cup, cooked) 8.85
Spinach (½ cup, cooked)...3.00

Sunflower oil (1 tbsp)..12.86
Sunflower seeds (¼ cup)..10.95
Sweet potato (1 med, baked)..7.80
Swiss chard (½ cup, cooked) 2.25
Thousand island dressing (1 tbsp)*...7.50
Tofu (½ cup)...6.30
Turnip greens (½ cup, cooked)...1.85
Walnuts (¼ cup) 1.35
Wheat germ (¼ cup, toasted) 11.66
Wheat germ oil (1 tbsp)..52.02
Wild rice (1 cup)...4.80

* The vitamin E content of most low-calorie dressings is substantially lower.

How Much Vitamin E Are People in the United States Getting?

The amount of vitamin E available in our food supply has increased dramatically during this century, with about two-thirds of our vitamin E intake now coming from fats and oils. Government statistics from the Continuing Survey of Food Intakes by Individuals (1985–1986) show that the average woman, for example, consumes 10.5 mg of vitamin E per day. While that approaches the RDA, consumption ranges widely among individuals, and many women actually had much lower intakes. (Those at the 5th percentile, for example, had intakes of only 3.75 mg per day.) Among women ages 19 to 50 years, 70 percent were getting less than the RDA of vitamin E.

How Much Vitamin E Are You Getting?

Before you decide that you need to take vitamin supplements or change the way you eat, you should know where you stand and how much improvement you really need. To help you analyze your current diet, we've developed a system you can use to calculate your approximate vitamin E intake. (You'll find this system in the other vitamin and mineral chapters, too.) Following is a list of common food sources of vitamin E, arranged according to the percentage of our Optimal Daily Allowance of vitamin E contained in them. From our ODA range for vitamin E of 100 to 400 IU, we have chosen the more conservative dose (100 IU) as a yardstick in preparing these guidelines.

To determine your average daily intake of vitamin E, start by keeping an accurate food diary for three or four days. The longer you keep the diary, the more accurate your calculations will be. Write down exactly what you eat and drink, together with an estimate of the serving size. Don't concern yourself with precisely how much vitamin E each food item contains; simply use the chart to find the food item and the percentage of the ODA that it provides. Then add up the percentages to see if you reach 100 percent each day.

If a particular item in your meals is missing from this list (it would be impossible for us to include every food item here), use the nutritional information on the food packaging. Most packaged foods are required to list their vitamin contents on the label.

After you've determined how much vitamin E you are obtaining from your diet each day, you can calculate whether you need to take supplements to reach the ODA. Remember that this chart uses 100 IU as the ODA, so if your ODA falls elsewhere in our recommended range (from 100 to 400 IU), you will need to take that into account when calculating percentages. An 8 ounce glass of milk provides 5 percent of an ODA of 100 IU, for example; if you've decided that your ODA should be 200 or 400 IU, that glass of milk meets only 2.5 or 1.25 percent of your optimal dose, respectively.

After you've determined how much vitamin E you are obtaining through your diet, you can calculate whether you need to take supplements to reach the ODA. Let's say that you determine that you are getting 20 percent of your vitamin E target of 100 IU through diet alone. You are consuming 20 IU of vitamin E in your diet (20 percent x 100 IU = 20 IU). To make up the difference, we would advise you to supplement your diet with 80 IU of vitamin E in tablet form (100 IU – 20 IU = 80 IU).

Because vitamin E is commonly sold in doses of 100, 200, 400, or 1,000 IU, you may have difficulty finding a supplement in the precise amount you want. We recommend that you come as close as you can to your target without combining or cutting up tablets to make the dose come out even. In the case we've described, for example, we advise going a little higher than your 80 IU needs, and taking a 100 IU tablet, which will more than meet your optimal requirements without posing any risks.

PERCENTAGE OF VITAMIN E ODA

(Based on an ODA of 100 IU)

5 Percent

Almond oil (1 tbsp)
Almonds (¼ cup)
Canola oil (1 tbsp)
Cottonseed oil (1 tbsp)
Filberts (¼ cup)
Hazelnuts (¼ cup)
Macadamia nuts (¼ cup)
Milk (8 oz)
Safflower oil (1 tbsp)
Salad dressing (1 tbsp)
Soybeans (½ cup, cooked)
Sunflower seeds (¼ cup)
Sweet potato (1 med, baked)
Wheat germ (¼ cup, toasted)

10 Percent

Corn oil (1 tbsp)
Soybean oil (1 tbsp)

30 Percent

Wheat-germ oil (1 tbsp)

Our Recommendations

HOW MUCH VITAMIN E DO YOU NEED TO ACHIEVE OPTIMAL HEALTH?

We advise that you consume 100 to 400 IU of vitamin E per day. This is several times higher than the RDAs.

WHAT SPECIAL CIRCUMSTANCES MIGHT AFFECT THE AMOUNT OF VITAMIN E YOU NEED TO TAKE?

If you take certain medications (such as particular anticholesterol drugs), have a diet high in polyunsaturated fatty acids, have certain chronic illnesses, smoke, or are pregnant or breast-feeding, you should move toward the high end of our recommended ODA range of 100 to 400 IU of vitamin E per day.

IS IT POSSIBLE TO CONSUME THE OPTIMAL AMOUNT OF VITAMIN E THROUGH DIET ALONE?

Practically speaking, it is almost impossible to consume an optimal dose of vitamin E through diet alone. The average individual has a dietary vitamin E intake far less than even the minimal ODA. Nearly everyone will find it necessary to obtain part of their vitamin E requirements through supplements.

FOLIC ACID

When you think of vitamins most critical to your well-being, folic acid may not be among them—unless you've been pregnant recently and discussed this nutrient with your obstetrician.

But folic acid, also sometimes called folacin, is suddenly getting attention. Studies in the 1990s have found that it can protect against neural tube defects (NTDs), severe birth abnormalities involving the brain and spine. Based on this persuasive research, the U.S. Public Health Service and the American Academy of Pediatrics now advise all women in their child-bearing years to consume at least 0.4 mg of folic acid per day in order to reduce the risk of having a baby with an NTD.

Information from this research has fueled new interest in folic acid, a B vitamin that was identified, synthesized, and named in the 1940s. It has also caused concern, since folic acid deficiency is common throughout the world, including in the United States, particularly among infants and pregnant women. This B vitamin is important to infants because it promotes cell replication and rapid growth. Pregnant women need extra folic acid not only to help their fetuses develop properly, but also because their bodies break down the vitamin at an increased rate.

Nor is a shortage of folic acid in the diet your only concern; even if you have enough of the vitamin, your body may not utilize it well. Such drugs as anticonvulsants (used by people with epilepsy) and birth-control pills can keep your body from properly metabolizing folic acid.

Basic Functions

• Folic acid, together with vitamin B_{12}, is necessary for the most fundamental of biochemical processes, specifically the creation of genetic material (DNA and RNA). It plays a critical role in the production and division of cells, and in tissue growth.

• Folic acid assists in the production of heme, the iron-containing substances in red blood cells.

Who's at Risk for Folic Acid Deficiency?

If you answer yes to any of the following questions, you have an above-average risk of developing a folic acid deficiency.

• *Are you pregnant?* Pregnant women frequently have folic acid deficiencies if their diets are not monitored carefully. Because the fetus draws folic acid from its mother to promote its own cell division and growth, the mother is at high risk. All pregnant women should have prescriptions for folic acid supplements.

• *Are you breast-feeding?* Because folic acid is lost in breast milk, the RDA for women in the first six months of nursing is for 100 additional mcg of folic acid per day; thereafter, according to the RDAs, nursing women should take an extra 80 mcg of folic acid.

• *Do you consume large amounts of alcohol?* The diets of people who drink excessive amounts of alcohol tend to be low in folic acid. In addition, alcohol appears to interfere with folic acid absorption.

• *Do you use medications such as trimethoprim (for urinary tract infections), anticonvulsants, or birth-control pills?* In particular, anticonvulsant medication such as phenytoin, phenobarbital, and primidone can interfere with the absorption of folic acid.

• *Do you have a malignancy?* Because cancer cells replicate quickly, they use up a lot of folic acid and cause deficiencies.

• *Do you have another nutrient deficiency—particularly of vitamin B_{12}—whose symptoms can mimic those of a folic acid deficiency?* Vitamin B_{12} is needed for the body to properly metabolize and use folic acid.

• *Are you an older person?* Older people in low-income groups or in institutions are especially likely to have diets deficient in folic acid.

Signs of Deficiency

Folic acid deficiency can produce anemia, characterized by over-sized red blood cells. Symptoms of anemia include weakness, head-aches, heart palpitations, and irritability. Other symptoms associated with folic acid deficiency are stomach upset and diarrhea.

Toxicity

In general, even high levels of folic acid are safe. There is no con-vincing evidence of side effects for doses of less than 15 mg a day.

In very large amounts, however, folic acid may interfere with the body's absorption of zinc. In addition, supplements of this B vita-min can mask the signs of a B_{12} deficiency. High levels of folic acid can interfere with diagnosis of a serious blood disorder related to a vitamin B_{12} deficiency (pernicious anemia). Delays in this diag-nosis can lead to serious and permanent nerve damage, including paralysis.

High doses of folic acid can also prevent anticonvulsant drugs from working, leaving users prone to epileptic seizures. If you have epilepsy and use folic acid supplements, be sure to inform your doctor.

Health Merits

Some of the most exciting news in vitamin research comes from studies of the connection between folic acid and the prevention of birth defects.

NEURAL TUBE DEFECTS

About 2,500 cases of NTDs occur in the United States each year; worldwide, the number is 300,000 to 400,000. These include cases of spina bifida (failure of the spinal cord's protective sheath to close) and anencephaly (a partially or completely missing brain).

Researchers have suspected for some time that vitamins might play a role in protecting against NTDs, but the most convincing evidence now relates specifically to folic acid.

• A seven-country study published in 1991 evaluated 1,817 women who had conceived a child with an NTD. For the study, each woman received supplements of either (1) folic acid, (2) other vitamins, (3) folic acid and other vitamins, or (4) a placebo. Those in the groups receiving 4 mg per day of folic acid (with or without other vitamins) had a 72 percent reduction in their risk of another NTD pregnancy. Those who took multivitamin supplements without folic acid or placebo were not protected against NTDs. The researchers in this study advised that "public health measures should be taken to ensure that the diet of all women who may bear children contains an adequate amount of folic acid."

• In a study by Hungarian researchers, published in 1992, more than 7,500 women planning to become pregnant received daily either (1) a multivitamin tablet containing 0.8 mg of folic acid (as well as 11 other vitamins, 4 minerals, and 3 trace elements) or (2) a supplement containing only trace elements. The women began taking supplements at least one month before they became pregnant and continued after conception until at least the second missed menstrual period. Most were getting pregnant for the first time. Researchers examined the outcomes of the pregnancies of the more than 4,000 women who conceived. Among those who had received trace-element supplements, six had fetuses with NTDs. By contrast, there were no cases of NTDs among those who had received supplements of folic acid and other vitamins. In analyzing other birth defects, researchers found similar results: congenital malformations occurred more frequently in the trace-element group (41 cases) than in the vitamin/folic acid supplement group (28 cases).

PRECANCEROUS LESIONS

Some researchers have looked at folic acid's possible role in preventing precancerous changes in the uterine cervix, a condition called *cervical dysplasia*.

• In a 1992 study at the University of Alabama, Birmingham, researchers measured blood levels of several vitamins and minerals, including folic acid, in 294 women with cervical dysplasia and 170 women without this abnormality. The scientists found that women with low levels of folic acid were at greater risk for cervical cancer from such known factors as cigarette smoking and infection with HPV (human papilloma virus, the virus that causes genital warts). Women with HPV were five times more likely to have cervical dysplasia if their folic acid levels were low than if they were high.

How Much Folic Acid Do You Need?

Your body's need for folic acid can fluctuate widely, depending on factors such as age and circumstances. More than any other single group, pregnant women require an elevated consumption of folic acid. The RDAs call for more than doubling of folic acid intake during pregnancy.

CARDIOVASCULAR DISEASES

Researchers have found that elevated levels of an amino acid called *homocysteine* increase the risk of coronary disease and stroke. Studies have shown that adequate amounts of folic acid can reduce homocysteine levels, while low intakes can produce high levels.

Optimal Daily Allowance

All men and women, no matter what their age, should consume 400 mcg of folic acid per day. Folic acid is critical for women of child-bearing age, and we believe the same optimal dose is important for preventing cervical dysplasia in older women, and in helping to reduce the risks of cardiovascular disease in both sexes.

Folic Acid Content of Common Foods

Food Item	Amount of Vitamin (in mcg)
Acorn squash (½ cup, baked)	19
Almonds (1 oz)	17

Artichoke (1 med, boiled) 54

Asparagus (6 spears, boiled) 88

Avocado, California (½ med) 56

Avocado, Florida (½ med) 81

Banana (1 med) 22

Beets (½ cup, boiled) 45

Black beans (1 cup, boiled) 256

Blackeye peas (1 cup, boiled) 356

Brie cheese (1 oz) 18

Broadbeans (1 cup, boiled) 177

Recommended Dietary Allowances

Infants

0–6 months ....25 mcg

6–12 months .... 35 mcg

Children

1–3 years .... 50 mcg

4–6 years ....75 mcg

7–10 years ....100 mcg

11–14 years...150 mcg

Male Adolescents and Adults

15+ years...200 mcg

Female Adolescents and Adults

15+ years...180 mcg

Pregnant Women

....*400 mcg

Lactating Women

first 6 months ....280 mcg

second 6 months ....260 mcg

Since these RDAs were issued, the U.S. Public Health Service has advised all women of child-bearing age to consume 0.4 mg of folic acid per day, considerably more than the RDA listed here. If you have had one NTD-affected pregnancy, you have a greater chance of having another such pregnancy; be sure to discuss your risk with your doctor if you are planning to become pregnant again.

Broccoli (½ cup, boiled)..54
Brussels sprouts (4, boiled)..47
Butternut squash (½ cup, boiled)..20
Cabbage, green (½ cup, boiled)..15
Camembert cheese (1 oz)..18
Carrot (1 med) 10
Cashews (1 oz)..20
Cauliflower (½ cup, boiled)..32
Corn (½ cup, boiled)..38
Cottage cheese, low-fat (1 cup) 28
Dates (10, dried)..10
Egg (1 lg, boiled) 24
Endive (½ cup, raw)...36
Figs (10, dried)...14
Garbanzo beans (1 cup, boiled) 282
Grapefruit (½ med)..15
Grapefruit juice (8 oz)..26
Great Northern beans (1 cup, boiled)..181
Green beans (½ cup, boiled) 21
Hazelnuts (1 oz) 20
Hubbard squash (½ cup, baked)..17
Kidney beans (1 cup, boiled)..229
Lentils (1 cup, boiled) 358
Lima beans (1 cup, boiled)..156
Liver, beef (3½ oz, braised)...217

Food Sources

Folic acid is present in green leafy vegetables, oranges, legumes, nuts, liver and other organ meats, and whole-wheat bread and other whole-wheat products. Some fortified, ready-to-eat cereals also contain folic acid.

Folic acid is water-soluble and sensitive to heat. Up to 50 percent of folic acid in foods may be lost in processing and cooking. Losses can also occur if foods are stored where they are exposed to bright light.

Liver, chicken (3½ oz, simmered) 770
Milk, low-fat (8 oz) 12
Navy beans (1 cup, boiled)...255
Oatmeal, instant (1 pkt)..150
Okra (½ cup, boiled) 37
Orange (1 med)...47
Orange juice, from concentrate (8 oz) 109
Parsley (½ cup, raw) 55
Parsnips (½ cup, boiled)..45
Peanut butter (1 tbsp)...13
Peanuts (1 oz) 29
Peas (½ cup, boiled)..51
Pecans (1 oz)..11
Pineapple juice (8 oz)..58
Pistachio nuts (1 oz)..17
Potato (baked, with skin)...22
Potato (baked, without skin) 14
Potato chips (1 oz)...13
Spinach (½ cup, boiled)...131
Strawberries (½ cup, raw)..13
Sweet potato (baked)...26
Tofu (½ cup, raw) 19
Tomato (1 med) 12
Tomato juice (6 oz)..36
Turnip greens (½ cup, boiled) 85
Vegetable soup, chunky (1 cup) 17
Whole-wheat bread (1 slice)...14
Yogurt, low-fat (8 oz)...25
Zucchini (½ cup, boiled) 15

How Much Folic Acid Are People in the United States Getting?

Government studies show that the average person in the United States consumes about 280 to 300 mcg of folic acid per day through diet alone.

How Much Folic Acid Are You Getting?

Before you decide that you need to take vitamin supplements or change the way you eat, you should know where you stand and how much improvement you really need. To help you analyze your current diet, we've developed a system you can use to calculate your approximate folic acid intake. (You'll find this system in the other vitamin and mineral chapters, too.) Following is a list of folic acid food sources, arranged according to the percentage of our Optimal Daily Allowance contained in them. Since half a cup of green beans contains 21 mcg of folic acid and the ODA for folic acid is 400 mcg, we've listed green beans in the 5 Percent category. (We have erred on the conservative side when rounding off percentages.)

To determine your average daily intake of folic acid, start by keeping an accurate food diary for three or four days. The longer you keep the diary, the more accurate your calculations will be. Write down exactly what you eat and drink, together with an estimate of the serving size. Don't concern yourself with precisely how much folic acid each food item contains; simply use the list to find the food item and the percentage of the ODA that it provides. Then add up all these percentages to see if you reach 100 percent each day.

If a particular item in your meals is missing from this list (it would be impossible for us to include every food item here), use the nutritional information on the food packaging. Most packaged foods are required to list their vitamin contents on the label.

After you've determined how much folic acid you are obtaining from your diet each day, you can calculate whether you need to take supplements to reach the ODA. Let's say that you determine that you are getting 50 percent of your folic acid target through diet alone. You are consuming 200 mcg of folic acid in your diet (50 percent x 400 mcg = 200 mcg). To make up the difference, we would advise you to supplement your diet with 200 mcg of folic acid in tablet form (400 mcg – 200 mcg = 200 mcg).

Folic acid is most commonly available in tablets of 400 mcg. Even if you need only 200 mcg, taking this 400 mcg supplement is fine; you'll more than meet your needs without any real risk.

PERCENTAGE OF FOLIC ACID ODA
5 Percent

Banana (1 med)
Butternut squash (½ cup, boiled)
Cashews (1 oz)
Cauliflower (½ cup, boiled)
Corn (½ cup, boiled)
Cottage cheese, low-fat (1 cup)
Egg (1 lg, boiled)
Endive (½ cup, raw)
Grapefruit juice, canned (8 oz)
Green beans (½ cup, boiled)
Hazelnuts (1 oz)
Okra (½ cup, boiled)
Peanuts (1 oz)
Potato (baked, with skin)
Sweet potato (baked)
Tomato juice (6 oz)
Yogurt, low-fat (8 oz)

10 Percent

Artichoke (1 med, boiled)
Avocado, California (½ med)
Beets (½ cup, boiled)
Broccoli (½ cup, boiled)
Brussels sprouts (4, boiled)
Orange (1 med)
Parsnips (½ cup, raw)
Peas (½ cup, boiled)
Pineapple juice, canned (8 oz)

20 Percent

Asparagus (6 spears, boiled)
Avocado, Florida (½ med)
Bran Flakes cereal (1 oz)
Corn Flakes cereal (1 oz)
Orange juice, from concentrate (8 oz)
Raisin Bran cereal (1 oz)
Turnip greens (½ cup, boiled)

30 Percent

Lima beans (1 cup, boiled)
Oatmeal, instant (1 pkt)
Spinach (½ cup, boiled)

40 Percent

Broadbeans (1 cup, boiled)
Great Northern beans (1 cup, boiled)

50 Percent

Kidney beans (1 cup, boiled)
Liver, beef (3½ oz, braised)

60 Percent

Black beans (1 cup, boiled)
Navy beans (1 cup, boiled)

70 Percent

Garbanzo beans (1 cup, boiled)

80 Percent

Blackeye peas (1 cup, boiled)
Lentils (1 cup, boiled)

100 Percent or More

Breakfast cereals, most (1 oz)
Liver, chicken (3½ oz, simmered)
Product 19 cereal (1 oz)
Total cereal (1 oz)

Our Recommendations

HOW MUCH FOLIC ACID DO YOU NEED TO ACHIEVE OPTIMAL HEALTH?

We recommend that both men and women take 400 mcg of folic acid per day. Women of childbearing years particularly need optimal doses of this vitamin.

WHAT SPECIAL CIRCUMSTANCES MIGHT AFFECT THE AMOUNT OF FOLIC ACID YOU NEED TO TAKE?

You should be particularly conscientious about consuming optimal amounts of folic acid if you are pregnant or may become pregnant. An optimal dose may also be important if you are an older person, take certain medications, consume large amounts of alcohol, have cancer, or are breast-feeding.

IS IT POSSIBLE TO CONSUME THE OPTIMAL AMOUNT OF FOLIC ACID THROUGH DIET ALONE?

In a typical day, you might consume two glasses of orange juice, one Florida avocado, one cup of boiled lima beans, and one serving of instant oatmeal—enough to meet the ODA of folic acid. The average person falls short of our optimal recommendation through diet alone, however. You may need to obtain part of your folic acid requirements through supplements.

VITAMIN K

Few people, even among those who know about vitamins, have heard much about vitamin K. Yet this vitamin plays a key role in some of the body's most important functions, including blood clotting.

Basic Functions

• Vitamin K is important to the clotting of blood. The liver uses vitamin K to manufacture several compounds, including the blood-clotting factor prothrombin.

• Vitamin K appears to be necessary for proper bone formation.

Signs of Deficiency

Vitamin K deficiencies are rare, largely because this vitamin can be produced naturally in the intestines. Even so, some people may be prone to deficits—for example, long-term users of antibiotics, which can destroy vitamin-manufacturing bacteria in the intestines. Newborns may also have a problem: bacteria have not

---

Forms of Vitamin K

Vitamin K is really a group of compounds. Two forms—K_1 (phylloquinone) and K_2 (menaquinone)—occur naturally: K_1 is found in foods, and K_2 is manufactured by bacteria in the intestinal tract. Vitamin K_3 (menadione) is a synthetic and more active form of the vitamin.

yet colonized their digestive tracts. Newborns receive an injection of vitamin K, typically before they leave the hospital, to prevent deficiencies. Older children and adults can compensate for any shortcomings in vitamin K production in the body with a proper diet.

When a deficiency does occur, the symptoms are abnormal blood clotting and an increased tendency to bleed, which might cause nosebleeds, as well as gastrointestinal, urinary, and intercranial bleeding.

Toxicity

Naturally occurring vitamins K_1 and K_2 are rarely toxic. The synthetic form—K_3—*is* potentially toxic, however. When consumed in excessive amounts, it has been associated with anemia, impaired liver function in people who already have advanced liver disease, and jaundice in infants. Jaundice is a yellowish coloring of the skin caused by the buildup of bilirubin, a by-product of the normal breakdown of red blood cells. Jaundice can lead to severe neurological problems, such as deafness and mental retardation.

Health Merits

Vitamin K helps the body manufacture the substances necessary for normal blood clotting. It also aids in the development of bones.

History

Much of our understanding of vitamin K dates back to studies done in Denmark in the late 1920s and 1930s. Dr. Hendrik Dam found that chickens on restricted diets bled spontaneously, and their blood clotted slowly if at all. Dam guessed that the deficiency-related condition had to do with a fat-soluble vitamin, and the problem did subside when the chickens received a particular fat-soluble nutrient. The initial *K*, for *koagulation* (the Danish spelling for the word that refers to blood clotting), was assigned to this substance.

How Much Vitamin K Do You Need?

Although vitamin K is not one of the better known vitamin, it does play an important role in the body. The RDAs for vitamin K are useful guidelines, and your needs for this nutrient can generally be met through dietary sources.

Optimal Daily Allowance

We recommend that you take 80 mcg of vitamin K per day as an optimal dose. We believe that this amount, at the high end of the range of RDAs, is ideal for both men and women.

Most people can obtain 80 mcg (and usually more) of K through diet alone. Single-dose vitamin K supplements are not widely available over the counter, but a few multivitamin preparations do contain small amounts of this nutrient.

Who's at Risk for Vitamin K Deficiency?

If you answer yes to any of the following questions, you (or your baby) have an above-average risk of developing a vitamin K deficiency.

• *Do you have a chronic illness (particularly a liver disease) or a disorder that interferes with the absorption of fats (such as ulcerative colitis, sprue, or Crohn's disease)?* These diseases can impair the body's ability to absorb and store vitamin K.

• *Are you a chronic user of mineral oil, anticholesterol drugs, or antibiotics?* The nonabsorbable fats of mineral oil attach to vitamin K and carry it out of the body. Some anticholesterol drugs (cholestyramine and colestipol) inhibit absorption of vitamin K. Certain antibiotics, including tetracycline, neomycin, and cephalosporins, suppress bacterial production of vitamin K.

• *Is your newborn breast-fed?* Because human milk is a poor source of vitamin K, breast-fed infants are more prone to deficiencies than infants fed fortified formula.

Vitamin K Content of Common Foods

Food Item	*Amount of Vitamin (in mcg)*
Asparagus (1 cup, raw)	52.26
Beet (½ cup, raw)	3.40
Broccoli (1 cup, raw)	116.16
Carrot (1 cup, raw)	17.81
Coffee (1 cup)	89.98
Corn oil (1 tsp)	2.73
Cucumber (½ cup)	3.50
Eggs (1 extra lg)	28.80

Recommended Dietary Allowances

Infants

0–6 months	5 mcg
6–12 months	10 mcg

Children

1–3 years	15 mcg
4–6 years	20 mcg
7–10 years	30 mcg

Male Adolescents and Adults

11–14 years	45 mcg
15–18 years	65 mcg
19–24 years	70 mcg
25+ years	80 mcg

Female Adolescents and Adults

11–14 years	45 mcg
15–18 years	55 mcg
19–24 years	60 mcg
25+ years	65 mcg

Pregnant Women

	65 mcg

Lactating Women

	65 mcg

Garbanzo beans (3½ oz, dry)...264.00
Green beans (½ cup)..15.40
Green cabbage (½ cup)...52.15
Green tea (1 cup) 1,686.02
Lentils (3½ oz, dry)...223.00
Lettuce (1 cup)..61.60
Liver, beef (3 oz.)...88.45
Liver, chicken (3 oz)...68.04
Liver, pork (3 oz)..74.84
Mushrooms (½ cup, raw)..2.80
Oats (½ cup)..25.42
Orange (1)..6.55
Peas (3½ oz, dry)..81.00
Soybean oil (1 tsp)..24.57
Soybeans (3½ oz, raw)..190.00
Spinach (1 cup, raw)...148.96
Strawberries (1 cup)...20.86
Tomato (½ cup)..20.70
Turnip greens (½ cup, raw)..148.75
Watercress (½ cup, raw)...6.63
Wheat germ (1 tbsp)..2.76
Whole-wheat flour (1 tbsp)..2.25
Yellow corn (½ cup, raw)...5.39

Food Sources

Bacteria in our intestines manufacture approximately half of the vitamin K we need. We must obtain the rest from our diets.

Spinach and other dark green leafy vegetables are among the best food sources of vitamin K. Significant amounts are also found in meat, milk and other dairy products, eggs, breakfast cereals, and fruits.

Vitamin K is not soluble in water and is quite resistant to heat during cooking. Exposure to light can destroy it, however.

How Much Vitamin K Are People in the United States Getting?

The U.S. Department of Agriculture and other sources estimate that, on average, people in this country consume adequate amounts of vitamin K. One study concluded that healthy adults consume an average of 300 to 500 mcg of vitamin K per day, well above the RDAs. Others suggest that this conclusion is high but that average intake is still at or above the RDAs.

How Much Vitamin K Are You Getting?

Before you decide that you need to take vitamin supplements or change the way you eat, you should know where you stand and how much improvement you really need. In fact, most people get all of the vitamin K they need through diet alone.

To help you analyze your current diet, we've developed a system you can use to calculate your approximate vitamin K intake. (You'll find this system in the other vitamin and mineral chapters, too.) Following is a list of vitamin K food sources, arranged according to the percentage of our Optimal Daily Allowance of vitamin K contained in them. Since 1 cup of raw carrots contains 17.81 mcg of vitamin K and the ODA for vitamin K is 80 mcg, we've listed carrots in the 20 Percent category. (We have erred on the conservative side when rounding off percentages.)

To determine your average daily intake of vitamin K, start by keeping an accurate food diary for three or four days. The longer you keep the diary, the more accurate your calculations will be. Write down exactly what you eat and drink, together with an estimate of the serving size. Don't concern yourself with precisely how much vitamin K each food item contains; simply use the chart to find the food item and the percentage of the ODA that it provides. Then add up all these percentages to see if you reach 100 percent each day.

If a particular item in your meals is missing from this chart (it would be impossible for us to include every food item here), use the nutritional information on the food packaging.

After you've determined how much vitamin K you are obtaining from your diet each day, you can calculate whether you need to take supplements to reach the ODA. Although most people meet or exceed the ODA of 80 mcg, you might find that you obtain, say, only 50 percent of your target through diet alone. That means you are consuming 40 mcg of vitamin K in your diet (50 percent x 80 mcg = 40 mcg). To make up the difference, we would advise you to supplement your diet with 40 mcg of vitamin K in tablet form (80 mcg – 40 mcg = 40 mcg).

Be aware that you might not find vitamin K pills sold in the precise dosage you need. In fact, while some health food stores sell vitamin K, most often in 100 mcg capsules, single-dose supplements of this vitamin are not readily available in some communities. Multivitamin supplements sometimes contain the amount of vitamin K that you will need, however; get as close as you can to the 40 mcg supplemental dose you need.

PERCENTAGE OF VITAMIN K ODA

5 Percent

Orange (1)
Watercress (½ cup, raw)
Yellow corn (½ cup, raw)

10 Percent

Green beans (½ cup)

20 Percent

Carrot (1 cup, raw)
Strawberries (1 cup)
Tomato (½ cup)

30 Percent

Eggs (1 extra lg)
Oats (½ cup)
Soybean oil (1 tsp)

60 Percent

Asparagus (1 cup, raw)
Green cabbage (½ cup)

80 Percent

Liver, chicken (3 oz)

90 Percent

Liver, pork (3 oz)

100 Percent or More

Broccoli (1 cup, raw)
Coffee (1 cup)
Garbanzo beans (3½ oz, dry)
Green tea (1 cup)
Lentils (3½ oz, dry)
Liver, beef (3 oz)
Peas (3½ oz, dry)
Soybeans (3½ oz, raw)
Turnip greens (½ cup, raw)

Our Recommendations

HOW MUCH VITAMIN K DO YOU NEED TO ACHIEVE OPTIMAL HEALTH?

We advise both men and women to consume 80 mcg of vitamin K per day.

WHAT SPECIAL CIRCUMSTANCES MIGHT AFFECT THE AMOUNT OF VITAMIN K YOU NEED TO TAKE?

If you have Crohn's or liver disease or ulcerative colitis or if you chronically use certain medications (antibiotics or anticholesterol drugs) or mineral oil, you may need to be particularly conscientious about consuming sufficient amounts of vitamin K.

IS IT POSSIBLE TO CONSUME THE OPTIMAL AMOUNT OF VITAMIN K THROUGH DIET ALONE?

Most people do consume vitamin K in amounts that meet or exceed our optimal recommendation.

CALCIUM

Calcium, the most abundant mineral in the human body, makes up about 2 percent of your body weight. About 99 percent of that is in the bones and teeth; the rest is in tissues and in the body fluids that bathe the cells. In order for your body to absorb the calcium from your diet and make use of it, you also need sufficient amounts of vitamin D.

A mechanism built into your body keeps the levels of calcium in your blood balanced—at sufficient but not excessive amounts. When calcium levels begin to rise too high, the thyroid manufactures a hormone called *calcitonin*, which draws excess calcium from the blood and deposits it in the bones; urine and feces also carry extra calcium out of the body. Conversely, when calcium levels dip too low, the parathyroid produces a hormone that pulls stored calcium from the bones and sends it to the blood. If the latter process goes on for too long, the bones are depleted of the calcium they need and become thin and weak.

Basic Functions

• Calcium is a key factor in building and maintaining strong bones and teeth. Even after their formation early in life, bones are continually rebuilt (or "remodeled"). Calcium is necessary throughout life, then—not just during the growing years of childhood and adolescence.

• Calcium controls the release of neurotransmitters (chemical messengers that pass impulses from one nerve to the next, carrying messages throughout the body).

• Calcium is necessary for muscle contractions. It is particularly important for the contraction of the heart muscle and the regulation of heartbeats.

• Calcium initiates the process of blood clotting by interacting with blood platelets and stimulating the proteins necessary for clotting.

• Some studies indicate that calcium may help regulate blood pressure.

• Calcium activates a number of enzyme systems in the body.

Who's at Risk for Calcium Deficiency?

If you answer yes to any of the following questions, you have an above-average risk of developing a calcium deficiency.

• *Are you an older person?* Older people do not absorb calcium as well as younger adults do and tend not to take in as much calcium to begin with.

• *Do you take diuretics?* Some diuretics change the function of the kidneys so that more calcium is lost in urine.

• *Do you exercise frequently?* Perspiration contains calcium. Your levels of this mineral can become depleted if you are extremely active physically—or if you exercise or perform physical labor in very hot weather—and you do not replace the calcium that you lose.

• *Are you on a low-calorie diet?* Dieting often cuts down on the intake of calcium.

• *Is your diet high in protein?* Individuals who eat lots of high-protein foods lose more calcium in the urine than other people do.

• *Is your diet high in fat?* Fats can bind themselves to calcium and interfere with its absorption.

Signs of Deficiency

If you do not take enough calcium, your bones suffer more than any other part of your body. Hormones work hard to ensure a balance of calcium levels in the blood, but that process can draw the mineral out of the bones, leaving them depleted and at potentially serious health risk.

The most common problem relating to long-term calcium deficiency is the disease *osteoporosis*, whose name means "porous bones" in Latin. In this condition, bones lack in substance and strength. Osteoporosis is most common in postmenopausal women, afflicting about 25 percent of females over the age of 60, but it also occurs in older men.

• *Is your diet extremely high in fiber?* Your body has more difficulty absorbing calcium if your diet includes a lot of fiber.

• *Are your vitamin D levels low—either because your diet includes too little vitamin D or because you have limited exposure to sunlight?* Vitamin D helps the body absorb calcium.

• *Is your diet high in phosphorus?* Foods rich in phosphorus—such as beef, pork, chicken, seafood, cheese, and nuts—may decrease the amount of calcium you absorb.

• *Is your diet high in phytates (found in whole grains) and oxylates (found in spinach, rhubarb, beet greens, and swiss chard)?* Both of these substances bind with calcium and keep it from being absorbed.

• *Are you pregnant?* A mother supplies an average newborn with about 30 g of calcium. As a result, the mother may be left with a deficiency.

• *Are you breast-feeding?* Breast milk contains 320 mg of calcium per liter. To replace this, mothers should take more of this mineral while nursing.

• *Are you a smoker?* Smokers have less bone density than non-smokers. Extra calcium may help to offset this condition.

The symptoms of osteoporosis can be devastating. A person might lose height when the vertebrae are deformed and collapsed, as in dowager's hump. Even more worrisome, the bones become increasingly fragile and brittle. A person with osteoporosis may suffer more fractures than a healthy person, not just from falls but from everyday activities such as lifting a child or a bag of groceries. These injuries may involve any bone in the body but are most common in the hip, spine, and wrist. Each year, about 1.3 million older people in the United States experience fractures related to osteoporosis.

While a calcium deficiency can certainly contribute to osteoporosis, other factors may also influence development of this complex disease. A scarcity of female hormones (estrogen), a chronic state of being underweight, and lack of exercise can all complicate matters.

Calcium deficits can affect parts of the body other than the bones, too. Low calcium intake might lead to modest increases in blood pressure, for example. A condition called *tetany*, in which a person experiences uncomfortable muscle spasms, has also been associated with severe calcium deficiency.

In children, poor absorption of calcium can produce rickets, a disease that stunts the growth of bones. (See chapter 10, "Vitamin D.") Symptoms of rickets include bowlegs, knock-knees, enlarged ankles and wrists, abnormal curvature of the spine, a bulging forehead, and a narrowed chest. In adults, deficits of calcium can lead to osteomalacia—frequently referred to as an adult form of rickets—which causes bones to soften and be more prone to fractures, deformities of the limbs and spine, and rheumatic-like pain.

Toxicity

Even large amounts of calcium generally do not pose particular risks for people. The natural workings of the body keep the blood levels of this mineral at a normal and safe level.

Very large intakes of calcium have at times been linked with certain health problems, however. Constipation, for example, has been reported in some people, particularly older people. So has the formation of urinary stones in men, as well as a decreased ability of the body to absorb zinc and iron.

In rare instances, very high consumption of calcium can overwhelm the mechanisms that maintain calcium balance. Excessive calcium can accumulate in the blood, producing toxic symptoms such as drowsiness, weakness, nausea, vomiting, and depression. In some cases, individuals may develop calcification of soft tissues, including the kidneys and other important organs.

Health Merits

OSTEOPOROSIS

Osteoporosis is a disease of declining bone mass, or density (the amount of material contained in the bone). Bone mass normally accumulates until a person is about age 25 and begins to deteriorate around ages 50 to 60 years; the bones then become weaker and much more vulnerable to fractures. Women experience a particularly rapid decrease in bone mass because of their sharp decline in estrogen levels during menopause.

You can take steps early in life to reduce your chances of having osteoporosis later on. The higher your bone mass is in your younger years, the less likely you are to develop osteoporosis, and the lower your chance of breaking bones. In other words, the more bone you start with, the more you can lose without running a risk of fractures. So one of the best ways to protect yourself against problems in later years is to consume enough calcium in your early years.

What about consuming calcium after your bones have stopped growing? In your forties, fifties, and beyond, how protective are large amounts of calcium? Experts disagree on the answers to these questions. Some insist that taking extra calcium during these years has little effect and that other factors (such as estrogen levels and exercise) are more important. We think, though, that calcium intake is crucial throughout life, helping to keep your bones dense, slowing bone loss, and preventing development of osteo-porosis. Some research supports this.

• A 1990 study was conducted at the U.S. Department of Agricul-ture Human Nutrition Research Center on Aging, Tufts Univer-sity, in Massachusetts. Researchers examined the possible effect of calcium on bone loss in 301 postmenopausal women—subjects who would normally be expected to lose calcium. The women received either (1) 500 mg of calcium carbonate supplements per day, (2) 500 mg of calcium citrate malate per day, or (3) a placebo. The researchers found that the women most likely to benefit from calcium supplementation were those who had little calcium in their diets before the study began. Women who had gone through menopause at least six years earlier significantly decreased their bone loss by increasing their calcium intake. Women who had gone through menopause five or fewer years earlier continued to lose bone rapidly, despite taking more calcium. In addition, researchers found that only calcium citrate malate supplements stopped spinal bone loss; both types of supplements halted losses in other parts of the body.

• In a 1992 study at Indiana University School of Medicine, re-searchers studied 45 pairs of identical twins, ages 6 to 14 years, for three years. One member of each pair took a 1,000 mg supplement of calcium citrate malate per day, while the other received a place-bo. Researchers intermittently measured bone densities in both groups. In prepubertal children, bone density increased in both supplemented and unsupplemented twins, but the increase was 1.4 percent greater in the supplemented group. There were no sig-nificant differences among older children.

• In 1992, French investigators examined 3,270 older women to determine how calcium and vitamin D supplements influenced bone fractures. During an 18-month period, half of these women took 1.2 g of elemental calcium and 800 IU of vitamin D per day; the other half received placebos. The women who received sup-plements had 43 percent fewer hip fractures during that time than those who took placebos. According to measurements taken at the beginning and end of the study, bone density in the women who took calcium and vitamin D supplements increased by 2.7 percent; it decreased by 4.6 percent in those who took placebos.

• In a 1993 study at Pennsylvania State University, researchers looked at the effects of calcium supplements on bone density in teenage girls. Ninety-four girls participated in the study; some took a daily 500 mg calcium citrate malate supplement, and the others took a placebo. Measurements at the beginning and end of the 18-month study indicated that bone density increased more in the girls taking supplements than in those taking placebos. These increases averaged an extra 24 g of bone (1.3 percent of the skeletal mass) annually during adolescent growth.

HIGH BLOOD PRESSURE

Although more research is needed, several studies have found that calcium supplements reduce blood pressure, at least in the short-term. This could affect a person's long-term chances of developing hypertension.

• In a 1984 study, detailed examinations of about 15,000 participants included a nutritional appraisal. Researchers found calcium to be one of the few dietary components consistently related to blood pressure readings. Higher levels of calcium in the blood were linked with lower blood pressure levels.

• In a 1986 study, Dutch researchers evaluated 90 men (ages 16 to 29 years) who had mild hypertension. Half of these men received 1 g of calcium per day for 12 weeks, while the others took a placebo. Systolic blood pressure did not change in either group; diastolic blood pressure, however, fell in both groups. (Systolic is the highest pressure, during heart contractions; diastolic is the lowest pressure, when the heart is relaxing.) This drop was significantly greater in the group receiving calcium supplements, with declines in that group averaging 4.5 mm Hg; the drop in the placebo group averaged 2.1 mm Hg. The 2.1 decline may have been due to a placebo effect—that is, the patients might have improved in their responses because they believed they had received an active treatment.

COLON CANCER

Some research has suggested a possible relationship between calcium consumption and colon cancer, although findings have not been consistent.

• In a 19-year-long multicenter study, researchers evaluated the calcium and vitamin D intakes of 1,954 men with and without colorectal cancer. According to the results, published in 1985, the noncancerous participants had taken roughly 10 to 15 percent more of these nutrients than the cancerous patients, suggesting that calcium may help protect against this type of cancer.

How Much Calcium Do You Need?

Not everyone agrees with the formal RDAs for calcium. A National Institutes of Health consensus panel on osteoporosis has advised that women consume more calcium than recommended in the RDAs—1,500 mg in the years after menopause if they are not taking supplemental estrogen. The National Osteoporosis Foundation recommends 1,000 mg per day for postmenopausal women who are not on estrogen replacement therapy.

Optimal Daily Allowance

Although the RDAs call for only 800 mg of calcium for men and women over the age of 25 (with an increase to 1,200 mg for pregnant and lactating women), we recommend a daily intake of 1,500 mg for everyone. Women clearly need more calcium to help protect them against osteoporosis, even if they are postmenopausal and on hormonal replacement therapy (which can also help protect their bones).

Men can benefit from extra calcium as well. According to some research, if men lived as long as women, the sexes would have similar incidences of osteoporosis. To be safe, men too should consume 1,500 mg of calcium per day.

Selecting Calcium Supplements

All calcium supplements are not created equal. As you browse through the supplement section at the health food store or pharmacy, read some labels. Calcium carbonate tablets (Os-Cal, Tums and others) provide a concentrated supply of calcium—40 percent pure calcium per tablet. Oyster shells are a source of calcium carbonate, so a label that says "oyster shell calcium" simply means that the product contains calcium carbonate.

When calcium carbonate makes contact with stomach acids, it is transformed into calcium chloride, which the body can easily absorb and utilize. People who have inadequate levels of stomach acid—a common condition among older people—may have trouble absorbing calcium, although taking calcium supplements with meals can help with this problem.

Supplements of other types of calcium—calcium citrate, calcium lactate, or calcium gluconate—have lower calcium concentrations: 24 percent, 13 percent, and 9 percent, respectively. Studies show

Recommended Dietary Allowances

Infants

0–6 months	400 mg
6–12 months	600 mg

Children

1–10 years	800 mg

Male and Female Adolescents and Adults

11–24 years	1,200 mg
25+ years	800 mg

Pregnant and Lactating Women

	1,200 mg

that the body absorbs calcium citrate more efficiently than any other form of calcium.

When choosing a form of calcium, stay away from dolomite or bone meal supplements. These supplements contain large amounts of calcium but can be contaminated with toxins such as lead.

Calcium Content of Common Foods

Food Item	Amount of Mineral (in mg)
Acorn squash (½ cup, baked)	45
Almonds (1 oz)	75
American cheese (1 oz)	124
Anchovy (3 oz, raw)	125
Apple juice, canned (8 oz)	16
Artichoke (1 med, boiled)	47
Asparagus (6 spears, boiled)	22
Beet greens (½ cup, boiled)	82
Black beans (1 cup, boiled)	47
Blackeye peas (1 cup, boiled)	42
Blue cheese (1 oz)	150
Brazil nuts (1 oz)	50
Brie cheese (1 oz)	52
Broadbeans (1 cup, boiled)	62
Broccoli (½ cup, boiled)	89
Brussels sprouts (4)	28
Buttermilk (8 oz)	285
Butternut squash (½ cup, boiled)	42
Cabbage, green (½ cup, boiled)	28
Camembert cheese (1 oz)	110
Carp (3 oz, raw)	35
Carrot (1 med, raw)	19
Cashews (1 oz)	13
Cheddar cheese (1 oz)	204
Clams (4 lg or 9 sm)	39
Colby cheese (1 oz)	194

Collards (½ cup, boiled) 74
Cottage cheese, low-fat (1 cup) 138
Crab (3 oz, cooked) 50
Crab (3 oz, cooked) 88
Cream cheese (1 oz) 23
Egg (1 lg, boiled) 28
Feta cheese (1 oz) 140
Figs (10, dried) 269
Flounder (3½ oz, raw) 61
Garbanzo beans (1 cup, boiled) 80
Gouda cheese (1 oz) 198
Grapefruit juice, canned (8 oz) 18
Great Northern beans (1 cup, boiled) 121
Green beans (½ cup, boiled) 29
Gruyere cheese (1 oz) 287
Hazelnuts (1 oz) 38
Herring (3 oz, raw) 49
Ice cream, vanilla (1 cup) 176
Ice milk, vanilla (1 cup) 176

Food Sources

People in the United States get most of their dietary calcium from milk and milk products such as cheeses. Since milk also contains vitamin D, which helps the body absorb calcium, milk is an especially good choice—whether whole, low-fat, or nonfat. (Milk producers call their product "fortified" because the vitamin D has been added.)

Other good sources of calcium include certain green leafy vegetables (such as broccoli and spinach), beans, nuts, and fish with edible bones (such as sardines and anchovies).

In addition to consuming foods that are naturally rich in calcium, look for products in your supermarket that are calcium-fortified. These include common items such as orange juice, breakfast cereals, and bread.

Kale (½ cup, boiled) 47

Lentils (1 cup, boiled) 37

Lima bean (1 cup, boiled) 32

Lobster (3 oz, cooked) 52

Macadamia nuts (1 oz) 20

Macaroni and cheese, homemade (1 cup) 362

Milk, low-fat, 1% (8 oz) 300

Monterey cheese (1 oz) 212

Mozzarella cheese (1 oz) 147

Muenster cheese (1 oz) 203

Mustard greens (½ cup, boiled) 52

Navy beans (1 cup, boiled) 128

Oatmeal, instant (1 pkt) 163

Okra (½ cup, boiled) 50

Orange (1 med) 56

Orange juice, from concentrate (8 oz) 22

Oysters (6 med, raw) 38

Parmesan cheese (1 tbsp, grated) 69

Parsnips (½ cup, boiled) 29

Peach (10 halves, dried) 37

Peanuts (1 oz) 17

Pear (10 halves, dried) 59

Peas (½ cup, boiled) 22

Pecans (1 oz) 10

Perch (3 oz, raw) 68

Pinto beans (1 cup, boiled) 82

Pistachio nuts (1 oz) 38

Pizza, homemade (1 slice) 144

Provolone cheese (1 oz) 214

Prune juice, canned (8 oz) 30

Prunes (10, dried) 43

Pudding, vanilla, homemade (1 cup) 298

Raisins, golden seedless (²/₃ cup) 53

Rhubarb (1 cup, raw) 266

Ricotta, part skim (½ cup) 337

Sardines, canned in oil (2)..92
Scallops (6 lg or 14 sm, raw)..21
Shrimp (12 lg, raw)...44
Sole (3½ oz, raw)..61
Sour cream (1 tbsp)...14
Spinach (½ cup, boiled)..122
Sunflower seeds (1 oz, dried)..33
Sweet potato (1 med, baked)..32
Swiss cheese (1 oz)...272
Tofu (½ cup, raw)..130
Trout (3 oz, raw)...36
Tuna, canned in water (3 oz)..10
Turnip greens (½ cup, boiled)...99
Wheat germ (¼ cup, toasted)...13
Yogurt, low-fat (8 oz)..415

How Much Calcium Are People in the United States Getting?

Most people in the United States consume less calcium than the RDAs. Women, who have a higher risk of osteoporosis than men, are more prone to deficits. They generally consume less calcium than men, averaging under 600 mg per day. A U.S. Department of Agriculture survey conducted in 1985 found that only 22 percent of younger women (ages 19 to 50) met the RDA for calcium consumption.

How Much Calcium Are You Getting?

Before you decide that you need to take vitamin supplements or change the way you eat, you should know where you stand and how much improvement you really need. To help you analyze your current diet, we've developed a system you can use to calculate your approximate calcium intake. (You'll find this system in the other vitamin and mineral chapters, too.) Following is a list of calcium food sources, arranged according to the percentage of our

Optimal Daily Allowance (1,500 mg) of calcium contained in them. Since 1 ounce of blue cheese contains 150 mg of calcium and the ODA for calcium is 1,500 mg, we've listed blue cheese in the 10 Percent category. (We have erred on the conservative side when rounding off percentages.)

To determine your average daily intake of calcium, start by keeping an accurate food diary for three or four days. The longer you keep the diary, the more accurate your calculations will be. Write down exactly what you eat and drink, together with an estimate of the serving size. Don't concern yourself with precisely how much calcium each food item contains; simply use the list to find the food item and the percentage of the ODA that it provides. Then add up all these percentages to see if you reach 100 percent each day.

If a particular item in your meals is missing from this list (it would be impossible for us to include every food item here), use the nutritional information on the food packaging. Most packaged foods are required to list their vitamin and mineral contents on the label.

After you've determined how much calcium you are obtaining from your diet each day, you can calculate whether you need to take supplements to reach the ODA. Let's say that you determine that you are getting 50 percent of your calcium target through diet alone. You are consuming 750 mg of calcium in your diet (50 percent x 1,500 mg = 750 mg). To make up the difference, we would advise you to supplement your diet with 750 mg of calcium in tablet form (1,500 – 750 mg = 750 mg).

Note that you may not find calcium pills sold in the exact dose you are looking for. We recommend that you get as close as you can to your target dose without taking several tablets just to get the precise amount.

PERCENTAGE OF CALCIUM ODA
5 Percent

American cheese (1 oz)
Anchovy (3 oz, raw)
Beet greens (½ cup, boiled)

Broccoli (½ cup, boiled)
Camembert cheese (1 oz)
Cottage cheese, low-fat (1 cup)
Crab (3 oz, cooked)
Feta cheese (1 oz)
Garbanzo beans (1 cup, boiled)
Great Northern beans (1 cup, boiled)
Mozzarella cheese (1 oz)
Navy beans (1 cup, boiled)
Pinto beans (1 cup, boiled)
Pizza, homemade (1 slice)
Sardines, canned in oil (2)
Spinach (½ cup, boiled)
Tofu (½ cup, raw)
Turnip greens (½ cup, boiled)

10 Percent

Blue cheese (1 oz)
Buttermilk (8 oz)
Cheddar cheese (1 oz)
Colby cheese (1 oz)
Figs (10, dried)
Gouda cheese (1 oz)
Gruyere cheese (1 oz)
Ice milk, vanilla (1 cup)
Monterey cheese (1 oz)
Muenster cheese (1 oz)
Oatmeal, instant (1 pkt)
Provolone cheese (1 oz)
Pudding, vanilla, homemade (1 cup)
Rhubarb (1 cup, raw)
Swiss cheese (1 oz)

20 Percent

Macaroni and cheese, homemade (1 cup)
Milk, low-fat, 1% (8 oz)
Ricotta, part skim (½ cup)
Yogurt, low-fat (8 oz)

Our Recommendations

HOW MUCH CALCIUM DO YOU NEED TO ACHIEVE OPTIMAL HEALTH?

We recommend an optimal intake of 1,500 mg of calcium per day for both men and women.

WHAT SPECIAL CIRCUMSTANCES MIGHT AFFECT THE AMOUNT OF CALCIUM YOU NEED TO TAKE?

You should be particularly conscientious about taking calcium if you are an older person, are pregnant or breast-feeding, exercise frequently, take diuretics, have a diet high in phytates or oxylates, or eat a low-fat, high-protein, high-phosphorus, or high-fiber diet.

IS IT POSSIBLE TO CONSUME THE OPTIMAL AMOUNT OF CALCIUM THROUGH DIET ALONE?

You can meet your optimal calcium needs by drinking three glasses of low-fat (1%) milk and eating two 8 ounce servings of low-fat yogurt per day, for example. Most people, however, consume less than half of our ODA through diet alone. You may find it more practical to get part of your calcium through supplements.

IRON

Having a deficiency in iron may at first seem rather implausible. After all, iron is plentiful in many foods we commonly eat—from red meats to vegetables to beans. In fact, though, this is the most frequent nutritional deficiency in the United States and throughout the world.

Why is this so? Part of the explanation is in the body's heavy demand for iron. Every cell in the body needs iron, which plays an important role in transporting oxygen. This mineral helps children and adolescents to grow. Women require iron for childbearing and for breast-feeding but lose a lot of the mineral through menstruation.

The iron you consume passes through the intestines and is absorbed by the bloodstream. About 70 to 80 percent of it ends up in *hemoglobin molecules*, which give blood its red color and which carry oxygen to cells throughout the body. Some iron also becomes part of a substance called *myoglobin*, a protein that supplies oxygen to muscle tissue.

Iron is found in other places as well. The liver, the spleen, and bone marrow store it in forms called *ferritin* and *hemosiderin*, for instance. But these stores can become depleted if you take too little iron over a long period of time. This is especially true for women who bleed heavily during menstruation or as a result of gynecologic abnormalities.

Who's at Risk for Iron Deficiency?

If you answer yes to any of the following questions, you (or your child) have an above-average risk of developing an iron deficiency.

• *Are you pregnant, or have you recently delivered a baby?* During pregnancy, the fetus and placenta demand a great deal of iron from your body. Blood loss during childbirth can also lead to an iron deficiency.

• *Are you menstruating?* The average woman loses 15 to 30 mg of iron each month during menstruation; women who bleed heavily or for long periods of time can lose significantly more. For this reason, women who have not yet reached menopause require more iron per day than men or older women.

• *Have you lost blood?* Gastrointestinal bleeding may occur with some conditions, including cancer, hemorrhoids, colitis, and ulcers. Blood loss can also take place during and after surgery or because of an injury. Aspirin or other nonsteroidal, anti-inflammatory drugs can also cause chronic bleeding.

• *Do you donate blood regularly?* You lose iron in every pint of blood you donate.

• *Is your diet rich in fiber or tea?* Each of these can interfere with iron absorption.

• *Are you a vegetarian, or do you eat little animal protein?* The body does not absorb the iron in foods in a typical vegetarian diet—including vegetables, beans, and grains—as easily as it does the iron in red meat.

• *Do you consume little vitamin C?* Vitamin C increases absorption of "nonheme" iron—iron found in plant foods. Even if you eat these iron-rich foods, your body will not necessarily absorb the iron from them unless you also consume enough vitamin C.

• *Are you taking antacids?* By altering the pH of the intestines, antacids can interfere with absorption of iron by the intestines.

• *Is your child young or an adolescent?* Children and teenagers need a lot of iron relative to their body size, partly because they grow so fast during this time.

Basic Functions

• Iron is important for transporting oxygen through the blood-stream. It enables hemoglobin to carry oxygen from the lungs to the body's cells.

• Iron is an essential part of myoglobin, the protein that stores oxygen reserves in muscles.

• Iron is present in a variety of enzymes and is important for critical reactions to occur inside cells.

Signs of Deficiency

Iron deficiency anemia is the most common condition related to inadequate amounts of iron in the body. With this form of anemia, the amount of hemoglobin in each red blood cell declines, reducing the oxygen-carrying capacity of the cell.

Babies and children with iron deficiency anemia often are pale, irritable, and hyperactive; have a short attention span; and lack energy. Adults may tire easily, feel listless and irritable, experience headaches, be short of breath, have a decreased appetite, and be more vulnerable to infections and illness. At the most severe stages of iron deficiency anemia, if the oxygen needs of vital organs are not met, this condition can result in a heart attack or a stroke.

Toxicity

If your health is generally good, you run little risk of experiencing side effects from high doses of iron (up to 75 mg per day), either in your diet or in supplements. People with an inherited disease called hemochromatosis *are* at risk, however. The intestines of people with this condition fail to regulate iron absorption properly, so the body tends to accumulate and store too much of the mineral. The extra iron can damage the body's most critical organs (including the liver, heart, and spleen) and bone marrow, causing serious problems like cirrhosis and irregular heart rhythms. Hemochromatosis tends to affect men more than women. Although this disease is rare, it can be deadly.

Excess Iron Intake: How Risky Is It?

In 1992, researchers conducting a study at the University of Kuopio, Finland, showed that excess iron in the body increased the chances of a heart attack. In fact, only cigarette smoking was more likely to lead to heart problems for men, according to the study.

During the three-year Finnish study, which involved nearly 2,000 subjects, men with blood ferritin levels of 200 mcg per liter or greater were more than twice as likely to have a heart attack as men with lower levels. Men who had both high iron readings and high levels of LDL ("bad") cholesterol were more than four times as likely to have a heart attack as men with low levels.

This study seems to support a theory proposed by Jerome Sullivan, a Veterans Administration pathologist, in the early 1980s. He suggested that the monthly loss of iron through menstruation in women before menopause might protect them from heart disease. After menopause, according to this theory, women had an increased risk of heart disease to correspond with increased levels of iron in the body after menstruation ended. Few researchers took this hypothesis seriously—until the Finnish study was published.

Although more recent research has raised doubts about the research at the University of Kuopio, the final word on this issue is certainly not out. In fact, a study published in April 1994 by the Center for Health Statistics, Center for Disease Control and Prevention, found contradictory evidence about the relationship between body iron levels (or "stores") and the risk of coronary heart disease. The study began in the early 1970s, when blood samples from over 4,500 men and women were used to determine body iron stores. Researchers followed subjects until 1987 to examine whether high iron levels were associated with an increased chance of heart disease. In this study, iron levels were not linked to heart disease. Furthermore in a somewhat surprising finding, iron appeared to have a *protective* effect.

Future studies should help clarify this issue. For now, it would be prudent to eat a diet rich in iron and to supplement it with low-dose iron tablets (up to 18 mg), if any. Only people with medical problems that cause chronic above-average loss of blood should take high-level supplements.

Children have a particularly high risk of iron toxicity. Thousands of cases of iron poisoning occur each year in youngsters, often after children swallow their parents' iron pills or multimineral supplements. An iron dose of about 3 g can be fatal for a child. (For adults, a fatal dose is estimated to be nearly 80 times higher.)

Health Merits

In addition to its role in normal body functions, iron is a specific treatment for anemia that results from chronic loss of blood.

How Much Iron Do You Need?

Note that the iron requirement for menstruating women is higher than for men and for postmenopausal women. Pregnant women have an even higher need.

Recommended Dietary Allowances

Infants
0–6 months ....6 mg
Children
6 months–10 years ....10 mg
Male Adolescents
11–18 years ....12 mg
Male Adults
19+ years..10 mg
Female Adolescents and Adults
11–50 years ....15 mg
51+ years..10 mg
Pregnant Women
....30 mg
Lactating Women
....15 mg

The dose of iron required to treat iron-deficiency anemia is much higher than the amount needed to maintain health. A typical recommendation for someone with iron deficiency anemia might include three 50 to 100 mg elemental iron tablets per day, often with vitamin C supplements to help absorption. This high dose of iron would be continued only until the anemia was corrected. If you have been diagnosed with this condition, though, do not immediately begin self-treatment. Ask your doctor for guidance.

On occasion, oral supplements do not end an iron deficiency. In that case, your doctor will probably recommend injections to bring your iron levels up to normal.

Optimal Daily Allowance

Our optimal dose guidelines for men are different than for women. We believe that the RDA for men (10 mg) is optimal.

Women, however, have greater needs for iron: at least 12 to 15 mg per day for optimal health. Those who bleed heavily during menstruation should raise the dose to 20 mg.

Iron Content of Common Foods

Food Item	Amount of Item (in mg)
Acorn squash (½ cup, baked)	0.95
Almonds (1 oz, dried)	1.04
Anchovy (3 oz, raw)	2.76
Apple juice, canned (8 oz)	0.92
Artichoke (1 med, boiled)	1.62
Avocado, California (½ med)	1.02
Bagel (1)	1.46
Beef, bottom round (3½ oz, braised)	3.25
Beef, brisket (3½ oz, braised)	2.19
Beef soup (1 cup)	2.32
Beef, top round (3½ oz, broiled)	2.81

Black beans (1 cup, boiled) 3.60
Blackeye peas (1 cup, boiled) 4.29
Brazil nuts (1 oz, dried) 1.00
Broadbeans (1 cup, boiled) 2.54
Broccoli (½ cup, boiled) 0.89
Brussels sprouts (4, boiled) 0.94
Carp (3 oz, raw) 1.05
Cashews (1 oz, dried) 1.70
Chicken breast (½, roasted) 1.04
Chicken leg (1, roasted) 1.52
Chicken, light and dark meat (3½ oz, roasted) 1.26
Chicken soup (1 cup) 1.73
Clam chowder, Manhattan (1 cup) 2.64
Clams (4 lg or 9 sm) 11.88

Food Sources

Popeye may have tried to convince us that spinach is the best food source of iron, but he was wrong. The body can better absorb the iron contained in many other foods.

Red meats (lean cuts) and liver are excellent sources of iron. Because of the high saturated fat and cholesterol contents of these foods, however, it is best not to rely on them too often.

Other excellent sources of iron are dark green leafy vegetables. Peas, corn, beans, dried fruits, prunes, and raisins are also good sources. In addition, many foods—including breakfast cereals, breads, and pasta—are fortified with iron.

Remember that your body will absorb iron from some foods better than from others. The best-absorbed iron—heme iron—comes from animal sources and can be found in meats, liver, chicken, and fish. The body does not absorb nonheme iron as well—iron from plant foods such as dried fruits, nuts, beans, and whole grains. Consuming meat, fish, or vitamin C (ascorbic acid) at the same meal with nonheme iron can help absorption. Vegetarians who eat only foods with nonheme iron have an increased chance of developing iron deficiency anemia.

Corn tortilla (1)..1.42
Corned beef (3½ oz, cooked)...1.86
Cream of Wheat (1 pkt, instant)..8.10
Dates (10, dried)..0.96
Egg (1 lg)..1.04
Figs (10, dried)..4.18
Flank steak (3½ oz, braised)..3.40
Garbanzo beans (1 cup, boiled)...4.74
Great Northern beans (1 cup, boiled).......................................3.77
Ground beef, lean (3½ oz, baked)..2.09
Haddock (3 oz, raw)...0.89
Ham, canned (3½ oz)...0.94
Hazelnuts (1 oz, dried)...0.93
Herring (3 oz, raw)...0.94
Kidney beans (1 cup, boiled)..5.20
Lamb, loin chop (1, broiled)...0.90
Leg of lamb (3 oz, roasted)..1.40
Lentils (1 cup, boiled)..6.59
Lima beans (1 cup, boiled)...4.50
Liver, beef (3½ oz, braised)..6.77
Liver, chicken (3½ oz, simmered)...8.47
Mackerel (3 oz, raw)..1.38
Marinara sauce (1 cup)..2.00
Mussels (3 oz, raw)..3.36
Navy beans (1 cup, boiled)...4.51
Oatmeal (1 pkt, instant)...6.32
Oysters (6 med)...5.63
Peanuts (1 oz, dried)..0.92
Peas (½ cup, boiled)...1.24
Pinto beans (1 cup, boiled)...4.47
Pistachio nuts (1 oz, dried)...1.92
Pita bread (1 pocket)...0.92
Potato (baked, with skin)...2.75
Prune juice (8 oz)...3.03
Prunes (10, dried)..2.08
Pudding, chocolate, homemade (1 cup)....................................1.30

Pumpkin seeds (1 oz, dried)..4.25
Raisins (²/₃ cup, seedless) 1.79
Rice, brown (1 cup, cooked) 1.00
Rice, white, enriched (1 cup, cooked) 1.80
Shrimp (12 lg)..2.05
Spaghetti, enriched (1 cup, cooked)..2.25
Spinach (½ cup, boiled)..3.21
Sunflower seeds (1 oz, dried)...1.92
Tofu (½ cup, raw) 6.65
Tomato juice (6 oz)..1.06
Tomato sauce (½ cup)...0.94
Trout (3 oz, raw)...1.62
Tuna, light, canned in water (3 oz)..2.72
Turkey, dark meat (3½ oz, roasted) 2.27
Turkey, light meat (3½ oz, roasted) 1.41
Turkey, light and dark meat (3½ oz, roasted) 1.79
Vegetable soup (1 cup)...1.63
Wheat germ (¼ cup, toasted) 2.58

How Much Iron Are People in the United States Getting?

The most recent government dietary statistics from the U.S. Department of Health show that certain groups of people are not meeting, on average, their iron RDAs. These include males from ages 1 to 18 years and females from ages 1 to 64 years. Women seem to be most susceptible to iron deficits: less than 20 percent of women between ages 9 and 64 years meet or exceed their RDAs.

How Much Iron Are You Getting?

Before you decide that you need to take iron supplements or change the way you eat, you should know where you stand and how much improvement you really need. To help you analyze your current diet, we've developed a system you can use to calculate your approximate iron intake. (You'll find this system in the other vitamin and mineral chapters, too.) Following is a list of iron food sources, arranged according to the percentage of our Optimal Daily Allowance contained in them. Our ODA for men is 10 mg; for women, it ranges from 12 to 15 mg, rising to 20 mg for women with heavy menstrual flow. For the purposes of this test, we have used an ODA of 15 mg.

To determine your average daily intake of iron, start by keeping an accurate food diary for three or four days. The longer you keep the diary, the more accurate your calculations will be. Write down exactly what you eat and drink, together with an estimate of the serving size. Don't concern yourself with precisely how much iron each food item contains; simply use the list to find the food item and the percentage of the ODA that it provides. Then add up all of these percentages to see if you reach 100 percent each day. Remember that we have based these percentages on an ODA of 15 mg; if your ODA is higher or lower, consider this in making your calculations.

If a particular item in your meals is missing from this list (it would be impossible for us to include every food item here), use the nutritional information on the food packaging. Most packaged foods are required to list their vitamin and mineral contents on the label.

After you've determined how much iron you are obtaining from your diet each day, you can calculate whether you need to take supplements to reach the ODA. Let's say that you determine that you are getting 60 percent of your iron target through diet alone. You are consuming 15 mg of iron in your diet (60 percent x 15 mg = 9 mg). To make up the difference, we would advise you to supplement your diet with 6 mg of iron in tablet form (15 mg − 9 mg = 6 mg).

Many supplemental pills contain 15 to 18 mg of iron, allowing you to meet—and perhaps exceed—your iron requirements with one pill, without any real risk.

PERCENTAGE OF IRON ODA
5 Percent

Acorn squash (½ cup, baked)
Almonds (1 oz, dried)
Apple juice, canned (8 oz)
Avocado, California (½ med)
Bagel (1)
Beet greens (½ cup, boiled)
Brazil nuts (1 oz, dried)
Broccoli (½ cup, boiled)
Brussels sprouts (4, boiled)
Carp (3 oz, raw)
Chicken, light and dark meat (3½ oz, roasted)
Chicken breast (½, roasted)
Chicken leg (1, roasted)
Chicken soup (1 cup)
Corn tortilla (1)
Dates (10, dried)
Egg (1 lg)
Haddock (3 oz, raw)
Ham, canned (3½ oz)
Hazel nuts (1 oz, dried)
Herring (3 oz, raw)
Lamb, loin chop (1 chop, broiled)
Leg of lamb (3 oz, roasted)
Mackerel (3 oz, raw)
Peanuts (1 oz, dried)
Peas (½ cup, raw)
Pita bread (1 pocket)
Pudding, chocolate, homemade (1 cup)
Rice, brown (1 cup, cooked)
Turkey, light meat (3½ oz, roasted)
Vegetable soup (1 cup)

10 Percent

Anchovy (3 oz, raw)
Artichoke (1 med, boiled)

Beef, brisket (3½ oz, braised)
Beef, top round (3½ oz, braised)
Beef soup (1 cup)
Broadbeans (1 cup, boiled)
Cashews (1 oz, dried)
Clam chowder, Manhattan (1 cup)
Corn Flakes cereal (1 cup)
Corned beef (3½ oz, cooked)
Flank steak (3½ oz, braised)
Ground beef, lean (3½ oz, baked)
Marinara sauce (1 cup)
Pistachio nuts (1 oz, dried)
Potato (baked, with skin)
Prunes (10, dried)
Raisins (²/₃ cup, seedless)
Rice, white, enriched (1 cup, cooked)
Shrimp (12 lg)
Spaghetti, enriched (1 cup, cooked)
Sunflower seeds (1 oz, dried)
Trout (3 oz, raw)
Tuna, light, canned in water (3 oz)
Turkey, dark meat (3½ oz, roasted)
Wheat germ (¼ cup, toasted)

20 Percent

Beef, bottom round (3½ oz, braised)
Black beans (1 cup, boiled)
Blackeye peas (½ cup, boiled)
Figs (10, dried)
Great Northern beans (1 cup, boiled)
Mussels (3 oz, raw)
Pinto beans (1 cup, boiled)
Prune juice (8 oz)
Pumpkin seeds (1 oz, dried)
Spinach (½ cup, boiled)

30 Percent

Garbanzo beans (½ cup, boiled)
Kidney beans (1 cup, boiled)
Lima beans (1 cup, boiled)
Navy beans (1 cup, boiled)
Oysters (6 med)
Raisin Bran cereal (¾ cup)

40 Percent

Clams (4 lg or 9 sm)
Lentils (1 cup, boiled)
Liver, beef (3½ oz, braised)
Oatmeal, instant (1 packet)
Tofu (½ cup, raw)

50 Percent

Bran Flakes cereal (¾ cup)
Cream of Wheat, instant (1 pkt)
Liver, chicken (3½ oz, simmered)

70 Percent

Clams (4 large or 9 small)

100 Percent or More

Breakfast cereals, most (1 cup)
Product 19 (1 cup)
Total cereal (1 cup)

Our Recommendations

HOW MUCH IRON DO YOU NEED TO ACHIEVE OPTIMAL HEALTH?

We recommend different amounts of iron as optimal for men and women. For men, we advise consuming 10 mg per day. Women should consume 12 to 15 mg per day. Women who experience heavy bleeding during menstruation should increase their daily intake to 20 mg.

WHAT SPECIAL CIRCUMSTANCES MIGHT AFFECT THE AMOUNT OF IRON YOU NEED TO TAKE?

You need to be particularly conscientious about taking your optimal amount of iron if you are pregnant or have recently given birth; you are menstruating or have experienced blood loss for other reasons, including donating blood regularly; your diet is rich in fiber or tea; you are a vegetarian or consume little vitamin C; or you take certain medications.

IS IT POSSIBLE TO CONSUME THE OPTIMAL AMOUNT OF IRON THROUGH DIET ALONE?

You can consume the ODA for iron solely through diet, but few people do. You may need an iron supplement if you want to reach your optimal intake for this mineral.

MAGNESIUM

If you eat lots of green leafy vegetables, whole grains, and legumes, you are consuming plenty of magnesium in your diet. That's good news, since a growing body of research suggests that an adequate amount of magnesium in your diet could promote a healthy heart, lower blood pressure, and more. Studies have shown, for example, that greater magnesium content in drinking water corresponds to a lower risk of heart disease, probably because magnesium decreases blood pressure.

Although every human cell needs magnesium, the body contains only an average of about 25 g of it. More than half of that is in the bones; the rest is in places like the teeth, the muscles, the soft tissues, and the blood.

Basic Functions

• Magnesium is important for many energy-dependent reactions to occur in the body.

• Magnesium is responsible for activating more than 300 different enzymes in the body. These enzymes are necessary for cells to function properly.

• Nerves require magnesium to function properly and to transmit impulses.

• Muscles need magnesium to act normally, particularly to relax. After calcium flows into muscles to help them contract, magnesium replaces the calcium and allows them to relax.

• Magnesium is a component of teeth and bones. It helps bones grow and plays a role in preventing tooth decay.

• Magnesium appears to help maintain a lower blood pressure.

Signs of Deficiency

Because magnesium is present in many common foods and in drinking water, few deficiencies of this mineral occur, particularly in healthy people.

Who's at Risk for Magnesium Deficiency?

If you answer yes to any of the following questions, you have an above-average risk of developing a magnesium deficiency.

• *Have you had a lengthy bout of diarrhea or severe vomiting?* Your body loses more magnesium during these episodes.

• *Do you consume large amounts of alcohol?* Magnesium deficiencies are common in alcoholics, primarily because of their poor diets.

• *Do you use diuretics?* Many diuretics cause magnesium to be lost in the urine.

• *Are you pregnant?* According to Recommended Dietary Allowances, pregnant women should take an additional 20 mg of magnesium per day. This is to meet the needs of the fetus as well as the increased needs of the mother because of her larger body (pregnant women gain an average of 30 pounds).

• *Are you breast-feeding?* Breast milk contains 30 mg of magnesium per liter; to replenish the magnesium lost in nursing, women should consume additional magnesium.

• *Does your parathyroid gland function poorly?* Hormones secreted by this gland help the body maintain normal magnesium levels.

• *Do you have diabetes or kidney disease?* People with these disorders excrete increased amounts of magnesium in the urine.

If you consume extremely low amounts of magnesium, however, you could experience nausea, muscle weakness or tremors, irritability, loss of appetite, gastrointestinal upset, and rapid heartbeat. Severe deficiencies may lead to confusion, disorientation, and coma.

Toxicity

If your kidneys are healthy, too much magnesium is not likely to cause serious problems. When your kidneys work properly, they can excrete any excess magnesium that you consume.

If you have diseased kidneys, however, excess magnesium can build up in the body and produce symptoms such as nausea, vomiting, and low blood pressure. In severe cases, more serious problems can develop, including troubled breathing, a slow heart rate, coma, and even death.

Health Merits

HYPERTENSION

Magnesium may help reduce high blood pressure. Some evidence suggests that too little magnesium in the body causes muscles in the blood vessel walls—the so-called vascular smooth muscles—to constrict. As the channels in these vessels become narrower, blood pressure tends to increase.

• In a study in Japan, reported in 1986, 21 men with high blood pressure received magnesium supplements of 600 mg per day. Researchers checked changes in the blood pressure of these patients and measured levels of magnesium in their red blood cells at the beginning and end of the four-week study period. As magnesium levels increased, blood pressure fell, with declines observed in both diastolic and systolic pressures during the course of the study. (Diastolic is the lowest pressure, when the heart is relaxing; systolic is the highest pressure, during heart contractions.)

• In a 1987 study of 615 men of Japanese ancestry, researchers with the Honolulu Heart Study examined the possible association between blood pressure and a variety of nutrients, including magnesium. Of the 60 factors they evaluated, dietary consumption of magnesium was most strongly linked to blood pressure control. As the men consumed more magnesium, their blood pressure readings fell.

• In 1993, Swedish researchers at Umea University Hospital studied 17 men and women with mild hypertension. Patients in one group received magnesium supplements, while those in the other group took placebos. The researchers monitored blood pressures in both groups over a nine-week period and then reversed the treatments—that is, those initially taking magnesium supplements received placebos for the next nine weeks, while those initially taking placebos took supplements. Blood pressure readings—both systolic and diastolic—fell substantially for the individuals in both groups when they took magnesium. The placebo produced no significant changes.

Although considerable evidence now supports magnesium's role in treating high blood pressure, not every study has found a positive effect upon hypertension.

• In a 1991 study at University Hospital, Uppsala, Sweden, investigators supplemented the diets of 71 men and women who had mildly high blood pressure with either magnesium tablets or placebos. Over a six-month period, some of these individuals—but not all—appeared to benefit from the supplements, with significant declines in blood pressure.

What's the bottom line? Many doctors believe that enough evidence exists for them to advise their patients with high blood pressure to eat foods rich in magnesium. The research continues.

HEART ATTACK

The studies are not yet conclusive, but magnesium seems to help save lives for patients who have just had heart attacks. Researchers believe that the mineral might relax the muscles within the blood vessels and thus improve blood flow, thereby helping heart-attack patients. Another theory is that magnesium somehow prevents heart muscle cells from suffering further injury.

• In a 1992 study, British researchers at Royal Leicester Infirmary injected more than 2,300 patients with either magnesium or a placebo soon after a heart attack. The patients given magnesium had a 24 percent greater chance of survival during the four-week period after their heart attack than those given placebos. Based on

Recommended Dietary Allowances

Infants

0–6 months	40 mg
6–12 months	60 mg

Children

1–3 years	80 mg
4–6 years	120 mg
7–10 years	170 mg

Male Adolescents

11–14 years	270 mg
15–18 years	400 mg

Male Adults

19+ years	350 mg

Female Adolescents

11–14 years	280 mg
15–18 years	300 mg

Female Adults

19+ years	280 mg

Pregnant Women

	300 mg

Lactating Women

first 6 months	355 mg
second 6 months	340 mg

these data, the researchers concluded that magnesium treatment could save an additional 25 lives for each 1,000 heart-attack patients treated.

OTHER DISORDERS

In ongoing studies, researchers are examining magnesium as a potential treatment for other health disorders, from osteoporosis to asthma to diabetes. To date, this research has been too limited to produce any conclusions.

How Much Magnesium Do You Need?

Because magnesium has many health-promoting functions, it is important to get enough of this mineral. Although the RDAs are designed to meet minimal requirements, optimal doses actually exceed the RDAs and help ensure that your body is maximizing the benefits of magnesium.

Optimal Daily Allowance

Because of the role magnesium may play in reducing heart disease and hypertension, this mineral is important for optimal functioning. We recommend a daily intake of 500 mg per day for both men and women. This dose is higher than the government's RDA, but we think the increase is important for maximizing magnesium's health benefits.

Food Sources

Many foods contain generous amounts of magnesium. The richest sources include nuts (particularly cashews and almonds), legumes, leafy green vegetables, and whole-grain cereals. (Note, however, that about 80 percent of the magnesium in cereal grains is lost when the germ and outer layers of the grains are removed during milling—so magnesium may be depleted in processed cereals.)

Except for bananas, fruits tend to be poor sources of magnesium.

Magnesium Content of Common Foods

Food Item	*Amount of Mineral (in mg)*
Acorn squash (½ cup, baked)	43
Almonds (1 oz)	84
Anchovy (3 oz, raw)	35
Artichoke (1 med, boiled)	47
Avocado, California (½ med)	35
Banana (1 med)	33
Beef, bottom round (3½ oz, braised)	23
Beef, brisket (3½ oz, braised)	18
Beef, top round (3½ oz, broiled)	30
Beet greens (½ cup, boiled)	49
Beets (½ cup, boiled)	31
Black beans (1 cup, boiled)	121
Blackeye peas (1 cup, boiled)	91
Brazil nuts (1 oz, dried)	64
Broadbeans (1 cup, boiled)	73
Broccoli (½ cup, boiled)	47
Buttermilk (8 oz)	27
Butternut squash (½ cup, boiled)	30
Carp (3 oz, raw)	25
Carrot juice (6 oz)	26
Cashews (1 oz)	74
Chicken, breast (½, roasted)	27
Chicken, leg (1, roasted)	26
Chicken, light and dark meat (3½ oz, braised)	23
Chicken, thigh (1, roasted)	14
Corn (½ cup, boiled)	27
Corn tortilla, enriched (1)	20
Crab (3 oz, cooked)	28
Dates (10, dried)	29
Figs (10, dried)	111
Flank steak (3½ oz, braised)	23
Flounder (3½ oz, raw)	30
Garbanzo beans (1 cup, boiled)	78

Grapefruit juice, canned (8 oz)..24

Great Northern beans (1 cup, boiled)..88

Ground beef, lean (3½ oz, baked)..17

Haddock (3 oz, raw)..33

Halibut (3 oz, raw)..71

Lentils (1 cup, boiled)..71

Ham, canned (3½ oz)..14

Hazelnuts (1 oz)..81

Herring (3 oz, raw)...27

Kidney beans (1 cup, boiled)..80

Lima beans (1 cup, boiled)..82

Liver, beef (3½ oz, braised)..20

Liver, chicken (3½ oz, simmered)..21

Lobster (3 oz, cooked)...30

Macadamia nuts (1 oz)...33

Mackerel (3 oz, raw)...64

Marinara sauce (1 cup)..59

Milk, low-fat, 1% (8 oz)...34

Miso (½ cup)...58

Mussels (3 oz, raw)..29

Navy beans (1 cup, boiled)...107

Okra (½ cup, boiled)..46

Orange juice, from concentrate (8 oz)..24

Oysters (6 med, raw)...46

Peanut butter (1 tbsp)...28

Peanuts (1 oz, dried)..51

Pear (10 halves, dried)...58

Peas (½ cup, boiled)...31

Pecans (1 oz, dried)..36

Perch (3 oz, raw)...26

Pineapple juice (8 oz)..34

Pinto beans (1 cup, boiled)...95

Pistachio nuts (1 oz)..45

Pork, loin (3½ oz, roasted)...19

Pork, shoulder (3½ oz, roasted)...18

Potato (baked, without skin)..39

Potato (baked, with skin)...55
Potato chips (1 oz)..17
Prune juice, canned (8 oz)...36
Prunes (10, dried)...38
Pumpkin seeds (1 oz, dried)..152
Raisins, golden seedless (²/₃ cup) 35
Scallops (6 lg or 14 sm, raw)...48
Sea bass (3 oz, raw)..35
Shrimp (12 lg) 31
Snapper (3 oz, raw)...27
Sole (3½ oz, raw) 30
Spaghetti, enriched (1 cup, cooked) 25
Spinach (½ cup, boiled)..79
Sunflower seeds (1 oz) 100
Tofu (½ cup, raw) 127
Tuna, canned in water (3 oz) 25
Turkey, light and dark meat (3½ oz, roasted) 25
Walnuts (1 oz)..57
Wheat germ (¼ cup, toasted) 91
Yogurt, low-fat (1 cup) 40

How Much Magnesium Are People in the United States Getting?

Recent surveys of the amount of magnesium in the typical U.S. diet are limited. A government study in the late 1970s concluded that about 75 percent of the people in this country regularly fell short of the RDAs for magnesium. Men of all ages tended to have more magnesium in their diets than women.

How Much Magnesium Are You Getting?

Before you decide that you need to take magnesium supplements or change the way you eat, you should know where you stand and how much improvement you really need. To help you analyze your current diet, we've developed a system you can use to calculate your approximate magnesium intake. (You'll find this system in the other vitamin and mineral chapters, too.) Following is a list of food sources of magnesium, arranged according to the percentage of our Optimal Daily Allowance contained in them. Since a Florida avocado contains 52 mg of magnesium and the ODA for magnesium is 500, we've listed the Florida avocado in the 10 Percent category. (We have erred on the conservative side when rounding off percentages.)

To determine your average daily intake of magnesium, start by keeping an accurate food diary for three or four days. The longer you keep the diary, the more accurate your calculations will be. Write down exactly what you eat and drink, together with an estimate of the serving size. Don't concern yourself with precisely how much magnesium each food item contains; simply use the chart to find the food item and the percentage of the ODA that it provides. Then add up all these percentages to see if you reach 100 percent each day.

If a particular item in your meals is missing from this list (it would be impossible for us to include every food item here), use the nutritional information on the food packaging. Most packaged foods are required to list their vitamin and mineral contents on the label.

After you've determined how much magnesium you are obtaining from your diet each day, you can calculate whether you need to take supplements to reach the ODA. Let's say that you determine that you are getting 40 percent of your magnesium target through diet alone. You are consuming 200 mg of magnesium in your diet (40 percent x 500 mg = 200 mg). To make up the difference, we would advise you to supplement your diet with 300 mg of magnesium in tablet form (500 mg – 200 mg = 300 mg).

Because magnesium is commonly sold in doses of 250 mg, and multivitamin tablets often supply 100 mg of this mineral, you may have difficulty getting a supplement of exactly the amount you want. We recommend that you get as close as you can to your optimal dose without taking several tablets just to get the precise amount, feeling free to go a little over the ODA without posing any real risks.

PERCENTAGE OF MAGNESIUM ODA

5 Percent

Acorn squash (½ cup, baked)
Anchovy (3 oz, raw)
Artichoke (1 med, boiled)
Avocado, California (½ med)
Banana (1 med)
Beef, top round (3½ oz, broiled)
Beet greens (½ cup, boiled)
Beets (½ cup, boiled)
Broccoli (½ cup, boiled)
Buttermilk (8 oz)
Butternut squash (½ cup, boiled)
Carp (3 oz, raw)
Carrot juice, canned (6 oz)
Chicken, breast (½, roasted)
Chicken, leg (1, roasted)
Cod (3 oz, raw)
Corn (½ cup, boiled)
Crab (3 oz, cooked)
Dates (10, dried)
Flounder (3½ oz, raw)
Haddock (3 oz, raw)
Herring (3 oz, raw)
Lobster (3 oz, cooked)
Macadamia nuts (1 oz)
Milk, low-fat, 1% (8 oz)
Mussels (3 oz, raw)
Okra (½ cup, boiled)
Oysters (6 med, raw)
Peanut butter (1 tbsp)
Peas (½ cup, raw)
Pecans (1 oz)
Perch (3 oz, raw)
Pineapple juice, canned (8 oz)
Pistachio nuts (1 oz)

Potato (baked, without skin)
Prune juice, canned (8 oz)
Prunes (10, dried)
Raisins, golden seedless ($^2/_3$ cup)
Scallops (6 lg or 14 sm, raw)
Sea bass (3 oz, raw)
Sesame seeds (1 tbsp, dried kernels)
Shrimp (12 lg, raw)
Snapper (3 oz, raw)
Sole (3½ oz, raw)
Spaghetti, enriched (1 cup, cooked)
Tuna, canned in water (3 oz)
Turkey, light and dark meat (3½ oz, roasted)
Yogurt, low-fat (1 cup)

10 Percent

Almonds (1 oz)
Avocado, Florida (½ med)
Blackeye peas (1 cup, boiled)
Bran Flakes (1 oz)
Brazil nuts (1 oz)
Breakfast cereals, most (1 oz)
Broadbeans (1 cup, boiled)
Cashews (1 oz)
Garbanzo beans (1 cup, boiled)
Great Northern beans (1 cup, boiled)
Halibut (3 oz, raw)
Hazelnuts (1 oz)
Kidney beans (1 cup, boiled)
Lentils (1 cup, boiled)
Lima beans (1 cup, boiled)
Mackerel (3 oz, raw)
Marinara sauce (1 cup)
Miso (½ cup)
Peach (10 halves, dried)
Peanuts (1 oz)
Pears (10 halves, dried)

Pinto beans (1 cup, boiled)
Potato (baked, with skin)
Spinach (½ cup, boiled)
Walnuts (1 oz)
Wheat germ (¼ cup, toasted)

20 Percent

Black beans (1 cup, boiled)
Figs (10, dried)
Navy beans (1 cup, boiled)
Sunflower seeds (1 oz)
Tofu (½ cup, raw)

30 Percent

Pumpkin seeds (1 oz)

Our Recommendations

HOW MUCH MAGNESIUM DO YOU NEED TO ACHIEVE OPTIMAL HEALTH?

We recommend an optimal intake of 500 mg for both men and women.

WHAT SPECIAL CIRCUMSTANCES MIGHT AFFECT THE AMOUNT OF MAGNESIUM YOU NEED TO TAKE?

Take extra care to meet your magnesium ODA if you are pregnant or breast-feeding; have diabetes, have parathyroid gland problems, or have had a lengthy bout of diarrhea or severe vomiting; are taking diuretics; or consume large amounts of alcohol.

IS IT POSSIBLE TO CONSUME THE OPTIMAL AMOUNT OF MAGNESIUM THROUGH DIET ALONE?

While you can, in fact, consume an optimal amount of magnesium in your diet, most Americans fall short. For that reason, the majority of people need to take magnesium supplements.

SELENIUM

Selenium is a late bloomer among minerals; not until 1979 was it described as a nutrient essential to human health. It is now classified as an antioxidant, with research suggesting that it could play an important role in preventing heart disease and certain types of cancer.

Basic Functions

• Selenium—in conjunction with an enzyme called glutathione peroxidase—acts as an antioxidant. In this role, it helps prevent oxidative damage in the body. In particular, selenium appears to

History

Until relatively recently, scientists had not uncovered clear evidence that selenium is an essential human nutrient. Finally, in 1979, researchers described an association between selenium deficiency and a heart-muscle condition called Keshan disease. The disorder, also called *cardiomyopathy*, affects primarily women in their childbearing years and children. Problems associated with it include cardiac enlargement and heart failure. In their investigations in the Chinese province of Keshan, researchers discovered that the soil there—and thus the diet of the people—was particularly low in selenium. They also learned that supplemental doses of 150 mcg of selenium per day could prevent Keshan disease.

work together with vitamin E to prevent injuries to cells. By consuming adequate amounts of both selenium and vitamin E, you can help your body fight off cell damage that can contribute to several serious diseases.

• Selenium appears to play a role in preventing heart disorders.

• Selenium seems to help prevent cancer.

• Selenium protects the body against the harmful effects of certain toxic substances, including arsenic, mercury, and copper. It appears to bind to these substances and render them less harmful.

Signs of Deficiency

A selenium deficiency may lead to symptoms such as muscular weakness and discomfort. In the most serious cases, selenium deficits can increase the risk of heart problems and cancer. Research suggests that the less selenium you have in your blood, the greater

Who's at Risk for Selenium Deficiency?

If you answer yes to any of the following questions, you have an above-average risk of developing a selenium deficiency.

• *Are you pregnant?* Women need extra selenium during pregnancy. According to RDAs, pregnant women should get an additional 10 mcg of selenium per day.

• *Are you breast-feeding?* Because about 15 to 20 mcg of selenium are lost in every liter of breast milk, RDAs advise that lactating women consume an additional 20 mcg per day of selenium.

• *Are you under physical or emotional stress?* Animal studies have shown that stress can contribute to selenium deficiencies.

• *Do you consume inadequate amounts of vitamin E?* To some degree, the roles of selenium and vitamin E overlap in the body. You may be able to make up for a deficiency in one of these nutrients by consuming more of the other.

your likelihood of developing coronary heart disease and having a heart attack. Many (but not all) studies have shown that greater selenium levels also correspond to lower incidence of cancer (such as lung, breast, urinary, and gastrointestinal cancers).

Toxicity

Too much selenium in the body can be toxic. Overdoses can cause symptoms such as nausea, abdominal pain, diarrhea, fatigue, irritability, a garlic-odor-like breath, and hair and nail damage.

Reports of selenium toxicity have been rare. According to one study, an individual developed toxic symptoms upon taking 1 mg per day over a two-year period. In another incident, a manufacturer mistakenly produced supplements containing 27 mg of selenium per pill. This pill produced toxic effects in more than a dozen cases.

Health Merits

Ongoing research into the effects of selenium has concentrated in two areas: cancer and heart disease. Findings indicate that selenium might help prevent both conditions.

CANCER

Research regarding prevention of cancer has produced conflicting findings. Although many studies suggest that high doses of selenium prevent the development of cancer, others are less conclusive.

The following studies suggest that high doses of selenium do help prevent cancer.

• In a large, multicenter study at universities throughout the U.S., reported in 1983, blood samples were collected from nearly 11,000 men and women. In the ensuing five years, 111 of these people developed cancer, and the selenium levels in their blood samples were compared to those of 210 cancer-free individuals. The amounts of selenium were substantially lower in the individuals with cancer;

people with selenium concentrations in the lowest one-fifth were twice as likely to develop cancer as those in the highest one-fifth. Cancers of the prostate and of the gastrointestinal tract were most strongly linked to low blood levels of selenium.

• In 1984, Finnish investigators at the University of Kuopio reported the findings of a study that examined a possible link between selenium and cancer. More than 8,000 men and women were interviewed, filled out questionnaires, and had their blood drawn and frozen. Over the next six years, 128 of them developed cancer. The blood samples of those 128 people were thawed and evaluated for their selenium content, as were the blood samples of 128 individuals who had remained cancer-free. The selenium levels were significantly lower in individuals who had developed cancer. Individuals with very low levels of selenium had three times the risk of contracting cancer (particularly of the gastrointestinal tract and of the blood) as those with higher levels.

• In a study reported in the Netherlands in 1993, more than 120,000 men and women completed dietary questionnaires and provided toenail clippings for researchers to use to determine their selenium levels. Over the next 3.3 years, 155 of these people developed stomach cancer, 313 contracted colon cancer, and 166 were diagnosed with rectal cancer. Although no evidence indicated that selenium might have protected the study population from either colon or rectal cancer, there was a suggestion that higher selenium levels reduced the risk of stomach cancer, particularly for men. Men ranking in the highest one-fifth of selenium levels had 36 percent less risk of developing stomach cancer than those in the lowest one-fifth.

Selenium levels do not appear to be associated with cancer risks for all types of cancer or in all cancer studies.

• As part of the Nurses' Health Study at Harvard Medical School, Cambridge, more than 62,000 nurses provided toenail clippings to researchers during 1982 and 1983. During the next 4.5 years, 434 of those women were diagnosed with breast cancer. The selenium levels in the toenails of the breast-cancer patients were found to be similar to the levels in the toenails of a similar number of cancer-free women—indicating no protection from the selenium.

CARDIOVASCULAR DISEASE

Studies such as the following indicate a link between selenium and cardiovascular disease.

• In a study that began in 1972, Finnish researchers froze blood samples from more than 11,000 men and women; they then followed those individuals for seven years. During that time, 367 of the participants developed cardiovascular disease; 170 died from the disease. Blood samples from the diseased individuals—and from an equal number of control individuals, without heart disease—were thawed and evaluated for their selenium content. The selenium levels were higher in the people who remained well. The individuals with very low amounts of selenium were about three times more likely to die of coronary heart disease—and twice as likely to suffer a heart attack—as people with high levels.

• In a 1984 study at Creighton University School of Medicine, Omaha, Nebraska, researchers examined the blood selenium levels of 91 men and women with chest pain, just before those people had x-rays taken of their coronary arteries (in a procedure called *arteriography*) to determine the presence and extent of their heart disease. In this study, the lower the selenium levels were, the more severe the coronary disease was. Individuals with disease affecting two or three of the arteries supplying blood to the heart had selenium levels significantly lower than those who did not have any apparent coronary artery disease.

• In a study at the University of Auckland, New Zealand, reported in 1990, blood selenium levels were determined in 252 men and women who entered the hospital because of heart attacks. Selenium measurements were also obtained from 838 healthy controls. Individuals experiencing heart attacks had selenium measurements about 6 percent lower than their healthy counterparts.

The half of the men who had lower selenium levels had a 60 percent greater risk of having a heart attack than the higher half; women in the lower half had a 70 percent higher risk.

How Much Selenium Do You Need?

Conclusive evidence of the need for selenium has emerged only in recent years, and our knowledge of this nutrient is still evolving. With some research indicating that elevated levels of selenium could help prevent certain types of cancer, we believe that the consumption of selenium at doses somewhat higher than the RDAs is important.

Recommended Dietary Allowances

Infants
- 0–6 months ....10 mcg
- 6–12 months .... 15 mcg

Children
- 1–6 years ....20 mcg
- 7–10 years ....30 mcg

Male Adolescents
- 11–14 years..40 mcg
- 15–18 years ....50 mcg

Male Adults
- 19+ years ....70 mcg

Female Adolescents
- 11–14 years..45 mcg
- 15–18 years ....50 mcg

Female Adults
- 19+ years..55 mcg

Pregnant Women
- ....65 mcg

Lactating Women
- ....75 mcg

Optimal Daily Allowance

We recommend that all people consume 100 mcg of selenium per day. This nearly doubles the RDA for women and is almost a 50 percent increase for men.

While you could probably safely increase your selenium intake to 200 mcg per day, it's unwise to go any higher because a few people may begin to experience adverse reactions at these elevated levels.

Selenium Content of Common Foods

Food Item	*Amount of Mineral (in mcg)*
Almonds (1 oz)	1.13
Apricots (4, raw)	1.48
Blackey peas (1/3 cup, boiled)	1.65
Brisket (3 oz, boiled)	2.55
Carrot (1 cup, raw)	1.37
Cashews (1 oz)	9.64
Celery (½ cup, raw)	1.80
Cheddar cheese (1 oz)	3.40
Chicken, dark meat (3 oz, roasted)	5.95
Chicken, light meat (3 oz, roasted)	5.10
Cottage cheese, low-fat (¼ cup)	2.26
Crab (3 oz, boiled)	14.46
Egg (1, extra lg)	3.15

Food Sources

Brazil nuts are the best dietary source of selenium. Seafood, liver, and kidney are also rich in selenium. Other meats tend to be good sources, too, as are milk and egg yolks.

Although grains and vegetables (especially mushrooms and onions) can contain substantial amounts of selenium, the precise level depends on the selenium content of the soil in which the crops were grown and the water used to nourish them.

Garbanzo beans (⅓ cup, boiled) 1.09
Grapefruit (½, raw)..1.20
Haddock (3 oz, steamed)..25.52
Ham, canned (3 oz)..6.80
Kidney beans (⅓ cup, boiled)...9.44
Macadamia nuts (1 oz)..1.98
Mushrooms (½ cup, raw)...3.15
Nectarine (1, raw) 1.37
Orange (1, raw) 1.31
Pecans (1 oz)..3.40
Pork chop (3 oz, grilled) 11.91
Salmon (3 oz, steamed) 18.71
Walnuts (1 oz)..5.39
Yogurt, low-fat (1 cup) 2.27

How Much Selenium Are People in the United States Getting?

Little data are available on selenium consumption patterns in the United States. One analysis, in the *Journal of the American Dietetic Association* in 1984, however, showed that the typical adult in this country takes an average of 108 mcg per day, well above the RDA.

How Much Selenium Are You Getting?

Before you decide that you need to take selenium supplements or change the way you eat, you should know where you stand and how much improvement you really need. To help you analyze your current diet, we've developed a system you can use to calculate your approximate selenium intake. (You'll find this system in the other vitamin and mineral chapters, too.) Following is a list of selemium food sources, arranged according to the percentage of our Optimal Daily Allowance contained in them. Since a 3 ounce serving of light chicken meat contains 5.10 mcg of selenium and the ODA for selenium is 100 mcg, we've listed this food item in the 5 Percent category.

To determine your average daily intake of selenium, start by keeping an accurate food diary for three or four days. The longer you keep the diary, the more accurate your calculations will be. Write down exactly what you eat and drink, together with an estimate of the serving size. Don't concern yourself with precisely how much selenium each food item contains; simply use the chart to find the food item and the percentage of the ODA that it provides. Then add up all these percentages to see if you reach 100 percent each day.

If a particular item in your meals is missing from this list (it would be impossible to include every food item here), use the nutritional information on the food packaging. Most packaged foods are required to list their vitamin and mineral contents on the label.

After you've determined how much selenium you are obtaining from your diet each day, you can calculate whether you need to take supplements to reach the ODA. Let's say that you determine that you are getting 60 percent of your selenium target through diet alone. You are consuming 60 mcg of selenium in your diet (60 percent x 100 mcg = 60 mcg). To make up the difference, we would advise you to supplement your diet with 40 mcg of selenium in tablet form (100 mcg – 60 mcg = 40 mcg).

Because selenium is commonly sold in doses of 50 or 100 mcg, you may have difficulty getting a supplement in the exact amount you want. We recommend that you get as close as you can without cutting up tablets just to get a precise amount. If you need a supplement of 40 mcg, it's fine to go a little higher and take a 50 mcg tablet to more than meet your needs without any real risk.

PERCENTAGE OF SELENIUM ODA
5 Percent

Cashews (1 oz)
Chicken, dark meat (3 oz, roasted)
Chicken, light meat (3 oz, roasted)
Egg (1, extra lg)

Ham, canned (3 oz)
Kidney beans (1/3 cup, boiled)
Walnuts (1 oz)

10 Percent

Crab (3 oz, boiled)
Pork chop (3 oz, grilled)
Salmon (3 oz, steamed)

20 Percent

Haddock (3 oz, steamed)

Our Recommendations

HOW MUCH SELENIUM DO YOU NEED TO ACHIEVE OPTIMAL HEALTH?

We recommend a daily intake of 100 mcg of selenium. Although a dose up to 200 mcg is acceptable, a few people may experience side effects from supplementation higher than 200 mcg.

WHAT SPECIAL CIRCUMSTANCES MIGHT AFFECT THE AMOUNT OF SELENIUM YOU NEED TO TAKE?

You should be particularly conscientious about consuming the ODA of selenium if you are under physical or emotional stress, take inadequate amounts of vitamin E, or are pregnant or breast-feeding.

IS IT POSSIBLE TO CONSUME THE OPTIMAL AMOUNT OF SELENIUM THROUGH DIET ALONE?

According to one survey, the average adult takes slightly more selenium than the ODA. Many people need a supplement to meet their optimal requirements, however.

ZINC

Except for iron, no other trace mineral is as prevalent in the body as zinc. And few have been as highly promoted. You may have heard a lot of claims about zinc, in fact; many myths have flourished around this mineral. Zinc has been touted as a treatment for angina, acne, liver disease, and lack of energy—despite scarce evidence to support any of these claims. Some proponents have even insisted that zinc stimulates sexual potency.

Setting aside the spurious claims, zinc *is* an essential nutrient that plays important roles in the body. It is present in all of the body's cells, with large amounts in the eyes, liver, bone, skin, hair, and nails.

Basic Functions

• Zinc helps promote the healing of wounds.

• Zinc is necessary for our immune defenses to function properly.

• Zinc is required for the efficient activity of many enzymes.

• Zinc is necessary for taste buds to function normally.

• Zinc is important in the normal physical growth of children. It is part of the structure of bones and is necessary for cells to properly form and remodel (or rebuild) bone.

• Zinc is an essential mineral for the normal functioning of the reproductive organs.

Signs of Deficiency

The effects of a zinc deficiency can be far-reaching. They include greater vulnerability to infections, poor healing of wounds, a loss of appetite, a poor sense of taste, skin rashes, and hair loss. Shortages of zinc can also slow normal growth in children, resulting in smaller stature and delayed puberty.

Who's at Risk for Zinc Deficiency?

If you answer yes to any of the following questions, you have an above-average risk of developing a zinc deficiency.

• *Is your diet high in fiber?* Dietary fiber can interfere with your body's absorption of zinc. Phytates, found primarily in whole grains and beans, particularly interfere with zinc absorption.

• *Does your diet contain large amounts of phosphorus or iron?* Although the research is not entirely clear on this point, some studies suggest that these minerals may mildly affect absorption of zinc. Phosphorus-rich foods include milk, meats, fish, poultry, and cheese. For a list of iron-rich foods, see "Iron Content of Common Foods" in chapter 15, "Iron."

• *Are you a strict vegetarian?* Because the vegetarian diet lacks certain types of food—particularly animal protein and milk products—you may consume less zinc than your body needs.

• *Are you pregnant?* During pregnancy, you need additional zinc to meet the needs of the placenta and the fetus. In animal studies, zinc deficiencies have been associated with developmental disorders in the young.

• *Are you breast-feeding?* Breast milk contains about 1.5 mg of zinc per liter; RDAs advise consuming an additional 7 mg of zinc per day in order to make up for this loss while breast-feeding.

• *Do you drink large amounts of alcohol?* Regular consumption of large amounts of alcohol can accelerate loss of zinc in the urine.

• *Are you an older person?* Some older people have poor diets that are deficient in zinc.

Low levels of zinc in a pregnant woman can put the fetus at risk, particularly during the latter stages of pregnancy.

Particularly prone to zinc deficiencies are people with sickle-cell anemia because their zinc-rich blood cells are broken down in large quantities, and the zinc thus freed is lost from the body through the urine. Whole-grain foods can also make it harder for your body to use the zinc in your diet. These foods contain substances called *phytates*, which attach themselves to zinc and block its absorption by the intestines.

Toxicity

Zinc does not generally cause toxic symptoms, except in very large amounts—such as 2 g or more taken at one time, or less (but still a lot) taken regularly over several weeks. By taking as little as two times the RDA of zinc over a period of months, for example, you can interfere with the status of copper in your body.

If you do have too much zinc in your body, you could experience vomiting and diarrhea, and have a decreased HDL ("good") cholesterol level. More serious problems include anemia and an impaired immune function. Very high zinc intake—10 to 30 times the RDA for prolonged periods—can interfere with your immune system (as can levels that are too low).

Health Merits

Zinc has been recommended for a variety of therapeutic uses, many of which have little or no scientific basis to support them. But zinc does appear to have some legitimate uses. Supplements of this mineral, in fact, may help your body fight off a variety of disorders.

IMMUNE FUNCTION

• In a 1981 study by Belgian researchers, 15 men and women over 70 years of age received zinc supplements every day for a month; another group of older subjects did not receive supplements.

Doctors monitored both groups for functioning of the immune system. After the month, the group taking zinc supplements had significantly improved in some aspects of their ability to fight disease; they had more circulating white blood cells, and their antibody response to the tetanus vaccine improved.

• In a 1981 study in Belgium, 83 men and women received supplements of zinc each day for one month; researchers then compared the immune systems of these people to those of 20 people who had not received additional zinc. Immune-system responses—such as the reaction of white blood cells to foreign substances (*mitogens*)— were significantly stronger after zinc therapy; responses did not change in the control group.

• A 1987 report from the Institute of Nutrition and Food Technology at the University of Chile described the effects of zinc supplementation on 32 infants recovering from modest levels of malnutrition. After researchers evaluated the immune systems of the infants, each infant received the same type of formula; half received additional zinc. Three months later, researchers re-evaluated the immune systems of the infants. Functioning of the immune system—including the response of white blood cells to foreign substances—improved only in the children who had received zinc supplements. Infants with the most zinc in their blood ran fevers for the least number of days.

How Much Zinc Do You Need?

Since potentially serious risks are associated with zinc deficiencies, you need to consume significant amounts of this mineral. These intake levels, which are above the RDAs, require zinc supplementation for many people.

Optimal Daily Allowance

Taking extra zinc has clear benefits, but the optimal range for this mineral is small. We recommend 15 to 25 mg of zinc per day; you do not need more than that.

Most people in the United States consume less than the ODA for zinc through diet alone and could benefit from supplementation. We often advise people to take daily supplements of 15 mg, which, together with the zinc from their foods, puts them at the upper end—or slightly above—our recommended range.

Zinc Content of Common Foods

Food Item	Amount of Vitamin (in mg)
Almonds (1 oz)	0.83
American cheese (1 oz)	0.85
Anchovy (3 oz, raw)	1.46
Bacon (3 pieces, fried)	0.62
Beef, bottom round (3½ oz, braised)	5.13
Beef, brisket (3½ oz, braised)	5.01
Beef soup, chunky (1 cup)	2.64
Beef, top round (3½ oz, braised)	5.40
Black beans (1 cup, boiled)	1.92

Recommended Dietary Allowances

Infants
0–12 months ....5 mg

Children
1–10 years ....10 mg

Male Adolescents and Adults
11+ years ....15 mg

Female Adolescents and Adults
11+ years ....12 mg

Pregnant Women
..............15 mg

Lactating Women
first 6 months ....19 mg
second 6 months ....16 mg

Blackeye peas (1 cup, boiled) 2.20
Blue cheese (1 oz)..0.75
Brazil nuts (1 oz) 1.30
Broadbeans (1 cup, boiled) 1.72
Buttermilk (8 oz) 1.03
Carp (3 oz, raw)...1.26
Cashews (1 oz) 1.59
Cheddar cheese (1 oz) 0.88
Chicken, breast (½, roasted) 1.00
Chicken, dark meat (3½ oz, roasted).......................................2.49
Chicken, leg (1, roasted)..2.96
Chicken, light and dark meat (3½ oz, roasted).......................1.94
Chicken, light meat (3½ oz, roasted).......................................1.23
Chicken soup, chunky (1 cup) 1.00
Chicken, thigh (1, roasted) 1.46
Clam chowder, Manhattan (1 cup)...1.68
Clams (4 lg or 9 sm, raw)...1.16
Colby cheese (1 oz) 0.87
Corned beef (3½ oz, cooked) 4.58
Cottage cheese, low-fat (1 cup)..0.80
Crab (3 oz, cooked)...3.58
Egg (1 lg, boiled)..0.72
Feta cheese (1 oz) 0.82

Food Sources

Most of the zinc in the average U.S. diet comes from animal products. The best sources of zinc include red meats, liver, and seafood. Egg yolks and milk are also good sources of zinc.

The amount of zinc contained in plants depends to some degree
on the soil in which the plants were grown, specifically on zinc
concentrations in that soil. In general, the best plant sources
include legumes such as blackeye peas. Although whole grains
are also good sources of this mineral, the body does not absorb
the zinc from them as well as from other sources.

Flank steak (3½ oz, broiled)...4.71
Gouda cheese (1 oz)..1.11
Great Northern beans (1 cup, boiled) 1.55
Ground beef, lean (3½ oz, braised)..5.10
Ham, canned (3.5 oz)..1.66
Hazelnuts (1 oz) 0.68
Herring (3 oz, raw) 0.84
Hot dog, beef (1) 1.24
Ice cream, vanilla (1 cup)..1.41
Ice milk, vanilla (1 cup)..0.55
Kidney beans (1 cup, boiled)..1.89
Lentils (1 cup, boiled)...2.50
Lima beans (1 cup, boiled) 1.79
Liver, beef (3½ oz, braised)..6.07
Liver, chicken (3½ oz, simmered)..4.34
Lobster (3 oz, cooked) 2.48
Macadamia nuts (1 oz)..0.49
Marinara sauce (1 cup)...0.67
Milk, low-fat, 1% (8 oz)...0.95
Monterey cheese (1 oz)..0.85
Mozzarella cheese (1 oz) 0.63
Muenster cheese (1 oz)..0.80
Mussels (3 oz, raw)...1.36
Navy beans (1 cup, boiled)...1.93
Oatmeal, instant (1 pkt) 1.00
Oysters, Atlantic (6 med)...76.40
Oysters, Pacific (6 med) 14.13
Peanut butter (1 tbsp)...0.47
Peanuts (1 oz) 0.93
Peas (½ cup, boiled)..0.95
Pecans (1 oz, dried)..1.55
Perch (3 oz, raw) 0.95
Pinto beans (1 cup, boiled) 1.85
Pork, loin (3½ oz, roasted) 2.62
Pork, shoulder (3½ oz, roasted) 3.59
Provolone cheese (1 oz)...0.92

Pumpkin seeds (1 oz, dried)..2.12
Ricotta, part skim (½ cup)...1.66
Scallops (6 lg or 14 sm, raw)..0.81
Shrimp (12 lg, raw) 0.94
Spaghetti, enriched (1 cup, cooked) 0.70
Sunflower seeds (1 oz, dried)..1.44
Swiss cheese (1 oz)..1.11
Swordfish (3 oz, raw) 0.97
Tofu (½ cup, raw)...1.00
Trout (3 oz, raw)..0.56
Turkey, dark meat (3½ oz, roasted) 4.16
Turkey, light meat (3½ oz, roasted) 2.04
Turkey, light and dark meat (3½ oz, roasted) 2.96
Vegetable soup, chunky (1 cup)..3.12
Walnuts (1 oz)..0.97
Wheat germ (¼ cup, toasted) 4.73
Yogurt, low- fat (8 oz)..2.02

How Much Zinc Are People in the United States Getting?

Government studies did not attempt to evaluate the amount of zinc in the typical U.S. diet until the mid-1980s. Surveys then found that many men and women were not consuming RDA levels of zinc. Men ages 19 to 50 years, for instance, took, on average, 94 percent of their zinc RDA; women in the same age range consumed, on average, 56 percent of their RDA. Only 73 percent of children ages 1 to 5 met the RDA for their age group.

How Much Zinc Are You Getting?

Before you decide that you need to take zinc supplements or change the way you eat, you should know where you stand and how much improvement you really need. To help you analyze your current diet, we've developed a system you can use to calculate your approximate zinc intake. (You'll find this system in the other vitamin and mineral chapters, too.) Following is a list of zinc food sources, arranged according to the percentage of our Optimal Daily Allowance of zinc contained in them. Our ODA ranges from 15 to 25 mg; we have used the low end (15 mg) in calculating these percentages. (We have erred on the conservative side when rounding off percentages.)

To determine your average daily intake of zinc, start by keeping an accurate food diary for three or four days. The longer you keep the diary, the more accurate your calculations will be. Write down exactly what you eat and drink, together with an estimate of the serving size. Don't concern yourself with precisely how much zinc each food item contains; simply use the list to find the food item and the percentage of the ODA that it provides. Then add up all these percentages to see if you reach 100 percent each day.

If a particular item in your meals is missing from this list (it would be impossible for us to include every food item here), use the nutritional information on the food packaging. Most packaged foods are required to list their vitamin and mineral contents on the label.

After you've determined how much zinc you are obtaining from your diet each day, you can calculate whether you need to take supplements to reach the ODA. Let's say that you determine that you are getting 20 percent of your zinc target through diet alone. You are consuming 3 mg of zinc in your diet (20 percent x 15 mg = 3 mg). To make up the difference, we would advise you to supplement your diet with 12 mg of zinc in tablet form (15 mg – 3 mg = 12 mg). If you've decided that your optimal dose falls somewhere besides 15 mg in our recommended range (15 to 25 mg), take that into account when calculating percentages.

Because zinc is commonly sold in tablets containing 10, 30, or 60 mg, you may have difficulty getting a supplement of the precise amount you want. We recommend that you get as close as you can to your target by using the supplements that are available. Many multivitamin and mineral tablets, in fact, provide about 15 mg of zinc, which might meet all of your ODA needs.

PERCENTAGE OF ZINC ODA
5 Percent

Almonds (1 oz)
American cheese (1 oz)
Anchovy (3 oz, raw)
Blue cheese (1 oz)
Brazil nuts (1 oz)
Buttermilk (8 oz)
Carp (3 oz, raw)
Cheddar cheese (1 oz)
Chicken, breast (½, roasted)
Chicken, light meat (3½ oz, roasted)
Chicken, thigh (1, roasted)
Chicken soup, chunky (1 cup)
Clams (4 lg or 9 sm, raw)
Colby cheese (1 oz)
Cottage cheese, low-fat (1 cup)
Egg (1 lg, boiled)
Feta cheese (1 oz)
Gouda cheese (1 oz)
Herring (3 oz, raw)
Hot dog, beef (1)
Ice cream, vanilla (1 cup)
Milk, low-fat, 1% (8 oz)
Monterey cheese (1 oz)
Muenster cheese (1 oz)
Mussels (3 oz, raw)
Oatmeal, instant (1 pkt)
Peanuts (1 oz)
Peas (½ cup, boiled)
Perch (3 oz, raw)
Provolone cheese (1 oz)
Scallops (6 lg or 14 sm, raw)
Shrimp (12 lg, raw)
Sunflower seeds (1 oz, dried)
Swiss cheese (1 oz)

Swordfish (3 oz, raw)
Tofu (½ cup, raw)
Walnuts (1 oz)

10 Percent

Beef soup, chunky (1 cup)
Black beans (1 cup, boiled)
Blackeye peas (1 cup, boiled)
Breakfast cereals, most (1 oz)
Broadbeans (1 cup, boiled)
Cashews (1 oz)
Chicken, dark meat (3½ oz, roasted)
Chicken, leg (1, roasted)
Chicken, light and dark meat (3½ oz, roasted)
Green Northern beans (1 cup, boiled)
Ham, canned (3½ oz)
Kidney beans (1 cup, boiled)
Lentils (1 cup, boiled)
Lima beans (1 cup, boiled)
Lobster (3 oz, cooked)
Manhattan clam chowder (1 cup)
Navy beans (1 cup, boiled)
Pecans (1 oz)
Pinto beans (1 cup, boiled)
Pork, loin (3½ oz, roasted)
Pumpkin seeds (1 oz, dried)
Ricotta cheese, part skim (½ cup)
Turkey, light and dark meat (3½ oz, roasted)
Turkey, light meat (3½ oz, roasted)
Yogurt, low-fat (8 oz)

20 Percent

Crab (3 oz, cooked)
Liver, chicken (3½ oz, simmered)
Pork, shoulder (3½ oz, roasted)
Turkey, dark meat (3½ oz, roasted)
Vegetable soup, chunky (1 cup)

30 Percent

Beef, bottom round (3½ oz, braised)
Beef, brisket (3½ oz, braised)
Beef, top round (3½ oz, broiled)
Corned beef (3½ oz, cooked)
Flank steak (3½ oz, broiled)
Ground beef, lean (3½ oz, baked)
Miso (½ cup)
Wheat germ (¼ cup, toasted)

90 Percent

Oysters, Pacific (6 med, raw)

100 Percent or More

Oysters, Atlantic (6 med, raw)

Our Recommendations

HOW MUCH ZINC DO YOU NEED TO ACHIEVE OPTIMAL HEALTH?

We advise that you set your Optimal Daily Allowance between 15 and 25 mg of zinc per day. This is more than most people in the United States are presently consuming.

WHAT SPECIAL CIRCUMSTANCES MIGHT AFFECT THE AMOUNT OF ZINC YOU NEED TO TAKE?

Your daily consumption of zinc should be near the high end of our ODA range (of 15 to 25 mg) if your diet is high in fiber, phosphorus, or iron or if you are a strict vegetarian; if you are an older person; if you are pregnant or breast-feeding; or if you drink large amounts of alcohol.

IS IT POSSIBLE TO CONSUME THE OPTIMAL AMOUNT OF ZINC THROUGH DIET ALONE?

It is possible to consume 15 to 25 mg of zinc per day through diet, but to get the minimum of 15 mg, you would have to consume 10 cups of Manhattan clam chowder, ten 8 oz servings of low-fat yogurt, or more than 11 oz of braised brisket, for example. Most people need supplements to attain their zinc goals.

WHAT OTHER MINERALS DO YOU NEED?

CHAPTER 19

W e've already looked in-depth at the most important health-promoting minerals: calcium, iron, magnesium, selenium, and zinc. But many other minerals play important roles within the human body and are essential to good health. Like all minerals, these nutrients originate in soil and water and end up in the plants and animals we consume. You need only small quantities of some (such as chromium, fluoride, and copper); these are called *trace minerals*. Your body requires larger quantities of others (such as phosphorus); these are called *macrominerals*.

Your body has a sophisticated monitoring system that helps you maintain the mineral levels you need. This internal mechanism tends to take the minerals from your foods, absorb what you need of each, and excrete the rest. If you take too little of a mineral, your body can absorb it more efficiently, helping to maintain our good health.

Sometimes, however, this internal mechanism misfires. Your body may retain too much sodium, for example, which causes blood pressure to rise. For that reason, you need to be familiar with the possible symptoms of mineral shortages or overdoses, even if they happen only rarely.

The following chart provides essential information on the most important functions and sources of these minerals, the symptoms that can occur if you take too much or too little of them, and our Optimal Daily Allowances (ODAs). The chart does not include some minerals (such as nickel, cobalt, silicon, tin, and arsenic), primarily because evidence that humans need them is limited and/or because health food stores and pharmacies generally do not carry supplemental forms of them. Even for those that are included, most of the ODAs coincide with the RDAs, since not a lot is known about optimal dosages of these nutrients.

Summary of Minerals

Mineral	Main Functions	Best Sources	Signs of Deficiency	Signs of Overdose	ODA
Chloride	Maintains fluid balance in the body	Salt, soy sauce, processed foods	Disruption of acid-based balance	High blood pressure	750-3600 mg
Chromium	Plays a role in the metabolism of glucose	Whole-grain cereals and breads, meats, cheese, beans, brewer's yeast	Impaired activity of insulin	None identified	200 mcg
Copper	Plays an important role in properly using iron	Organ meats, shellfish, seeds, nuts	Anemia, bone abnormalities	Diarrhea, vomiting	1.5–3.0 mg
Fluoride	Promotes normal tooth and bone formation	Fluoridated drinking water, tea, milk, fish (if eaten with bones, such as anchovies and sardines)	Tooth decay	Mottling and pitting of teeth	1.5–4.0 mg

Mineral	Main Functions	Best Sources	Signs of Deficiency	Signs of Overdose	ODA
Iodine	As a component of thyroid hormone, contributes to metabolic processes throughout the body	Seafoods, iodized salt, vegetables grown in iodine-rich soil	Simple goiter (enlargement of the thyroid)	Simple goiter (enlargement of the thyroid)	150-200 mcg
Manganese	Assists in enzyme reactions	Whole grain cereals and breads, legumes, nuts	None identified	Nerve disorders (rare)	2.0–5.0 mg
Molybdenum	Assists in enzyme reactions	Whole-grain cereals and breads, milk, vegetables	None identified	Joint pain, copper deficiency	75–250 mcg
Phosphorus	Strengthens the bones and teeth, regulates enzymes and energy production, helps in the formation of cell membranes	Milk, meats, fish, poultry, eggs, cheese, legumes, whole-grain cereals and breads, nuts	Stunted growth, malformed and painful bones (rickets), weakness, loss of appetite	Reduced blood calcium levels, impairment of bone mineralization	800–1200 mg

Mineral	Main Functions	Best Sources	Signs of Deficiency	Signs of Overdose	ODA
Potassium	Maintains fluid balance in the cells, helps conduct nerve impulses and contract muscles, helps maintain normal blood pressure	Citrus and dried fruits, vegetables, legumes, milk	Muscle weakness, drowsiness, irregular heartbeat, loss of appetite, nausea, vomiting, irritability	Irregular heartbeat	2000-3500 mg
Sodium	Helps maintain a balance of fluids	Salt, processed foods	Headaches, muscle cramps, weakness	High blood pressure	500-2400 mg
Sulfur	Serves as a component of certain amino acids and vitamins	Peas, beans, wheat germ, poultry, beef, eggs	None identified	None identified	

* The ODA for this mineral is still undetermined, but most people get all the sulfur they need from their diet.

Vitamin Strategy Planner

Nutrient (Vitamins)	ODA	Your Personal ODA	Amount Obtained Through Diet	Amount Needed From Supplements
Beta-carotene	6–30 mg			
Biotin	30–100 mcg			
Folic acid	400 mcg			
Niacin (Vitamin B$_3$)	20 mg			
Pantothenic Acid	4–7 mg			
Riboflavin	1.8 mg			
Thiamin	1.5 mg			

Vitamin Strategy Planner

Nutrient (Vitamins)	ODA	Your Personal ODA	Amount Obtained Through Diet	Amount Needed From Supplements
Vitamin A	1,000 mcg RE (5,000 IU)			
Vitamin B₆	4 mg			
Vitamin B₁₂	5 mcg			
Vitamin C	250–1,000 mg			
Vitamin D	400 IU			
Vitamin E	100–400 IU			
Vitamin K	80 mcg			

Vitamin Strategy Planner

Nutrient (Minerals)	ODA	Your Personal ODA	Amount Obtained Through Diet	Amount Needed From Supplements
Calcium	1,500 mg			
Chromium	200 mcg			
Iron	10 mg for men; 15 mg for women; 20 mg for women with heavy periods			
Magnesium	500 mg			
Selenium	200 mcg			
Zinc	15–25 mg			

AFTERWORD

The benefits of vitamins and minerals are no longer speculative. The evidence is clear: these important nutrients—taken in proper quantities—can improve your chance of living a longer, healthier life.

As you incorporate optimal daily doses of each vitamin and mineral into your life—through a good diet and appropriate supplementation—keep in mind that research in this area is moving rapidly. Some of today's studies may be obsolete by tomorrow. We strongly encourage you to stay as informed as possible, using reliable sources of new data to keep up-to-date.

We also hope you will work with your physician to develop the nutritional program best suited to your specific lifestyle and medical needs. No book can replace the guidance of a health professional who is familiar with your unique health circumstances.

We hope this book helps you to achieve an optimum level of well-being. We wish you good health always.

—Art Ulene, M.D.
—Val Ulene, M.D.

BIBLIOGRAPHY

GENERAL

Holland, B., Welch, A.A., Unwin, I.D., et al. *McCance and Widdowson's: The Composition of Foods*. 5th ed. Cambridge, United Kingdom: The Royal Society of Chemistry, 1991.

National Research Council. *Recommended Dietary Allowances* 10th Edition. Washington, D.C.: National Academy Press, 1989.

Pennington, J.A. *Bowes and Church's: Food Values of Portions Commonly Used*. 15th ed. Philadelphia, PA: J.B. Lippincott Company, 1989.

VITAMIN A

The Alpha-Tocopherol, Beta-Carotene Cancer Prevention Study Group. "The Effect of Vitamin E and Beta-Carotene on the Incidence of Lung Cancer and Other Cancers in Male Smokers." *NEJM* 330 (1994): 1029-1035.

Blot, W.J., Li, J.Y., Taylor, P.R., et al. "Nutrition Intervention Trials in Linxian, China: Supplementation With Specific Vitamin/Mineral Combinations, Cancer Incidence, and Disease-Specific Mortality in the General Population." *Journal of the National Cancer Institute* 85 (1993): 1483-1492.

Comstock, G.W., Helzlsouer, K.J., Bush, T.L. "Prediagnostic Serum Levels of Carotenoids and Vitamin E as Related to Subsequent Cancer in Washington County, Maryland." *American Journal of Clinical Nutrition* 53 (1991): 260S-264S.

Connett, J.E., Kuller, L.H., Kjelsberg, M.O., et al. "Relationship Between Carotenoids and Cancer: The Multiple Risk Factor Intervention Trial Study." *Cancer* 64 (1989): 126-134.

Eye Disease Case-Control Study Group. "Antioxidant Status and Neovascular Age-Related Macular Degeneration." *Archives of Ophthalmology* 111 (1993): 104-109.

Garewal, H.S. "Potential Role of Beta-Carotene in Prevention of Oral Cancer." *American Journal of Clinical Nutrition* 53 (1991): 294S-297S.

Gaziano, J.M., Manson, J.E., Branch, L.G., et al. "Dietary Beta-Carotene and Decreased Cardiovascular Mortality in an Elderly Cohort." (abst) *JACC* 19 (1992): 377.

Gaziano, J.M., Manson, J.E., Ridker, P.M., et al. "Beta-Carotene Therapy for Chronic Stable Angina." (abst) *Circulation* 82 (1990): 201.

Jacques, P.F., Chylack, L.T. "Epidemiologic Evidence of a Role for the Antioxidant Vitamins and Carotenoids in Cataract Prevention." *American Journal of Clinical Nutrition* 53 (1991): 352S-355S.

Knekt, P., Heliovaara, M., Rissanen, A., et al. "Serum Antioxidant Vitamins and Risk of Cataract." *British Medical Journal* 305 (1992): 1392-1394.

Knekt, P., Jarvinen, R., Seppanen, R., et al. "Dietary Antioxidants and the Risk of Lung Cancer." *American Journal of Epidemiology* 134 (1991): 471-479.

Manson, J.E., Stampfer, M.J., Willett, W.C., et al. "A Prospective Study of Antioxidant Vitamins and Incidence of Coronary Heart Disease in Women." (abst) *Circulation* 84 (1991): 546.

Mayne, S.T., Jamerich, D.T., Greenwald, P., et al. "Dietary Beta-Carotene and Lung Cancer Risk in US Nonsmokers." *Journal of the National Cancer* Institute 86 (1994): 33-38.

Semba, R.D., Graham, N.M., Caiaffa, W.T., et al. "Increased Mortality Associated With Vitamin A Deficiency During Human Immunodeficiency Virus Type 1 Infection." *Archives of Internal Medicine* 153 (1993): 2149-2154.

Shekelle, R.B., Liu, S., Raynor, W.J., et al. "Dietary Vitamin A and Risk of Cancer in the Western Electric Study." *Lancet* 2 (1981): 1185-1190.

Stahelin, H.B., Gey, K.F., Eichholzer, M., et al. "Beta-Carotene and Cancer Prevention: The Basel Study." *American Journal of Clinical Nutrition* 53 (1991): 265S-269S.

Verreault, R., Chu, J., Mandelson, M., et al. "A Case-Control Study of Diet and Invasive Cervical Cancer." *International Journal of Cancer* 43 (1989): 1050-1054.

Wald, N.J., Boreham, J., Hayward, J.L., et al. "Plasma Retinol, Beta-Carotene, and Vitamin E Levels in Relation to the Future Risk of Breast Cancer." *British Journal of Cancer* 49 (1984): 321-324.

B₃ (NIACIN)

Coronary Drug Project Research Group. "Clofibrate and Niacin in Coronary Heart Disease." *JAMA* 231 (1975): 360-381.

VITAMIN B₁₂

Ubbink, J.B., Vermaak, W.J., van der Merwe, A., et al. "Vitamin B_{12}, Vitamin B_6, and Folate Nutritional Status in Men with Hyperhomocysteinemia." *American Journal of Clinical Nutrition* 57 (1993): 47-53.

VITAMIN C

Block, G. "Vitamin C and Cancer Prevention: The Epidemiologic Evidence." *American Journal of Clinical Nutrition* 53 (1991): 270S-282S.

Enstrom, J.E., Kanim, L.E., Klein, M.A. "Vitamin C Intake and Mortality Among a Sample of the US Population." *Epidemiology* 3 (1992): 194-202.

Howe, G.R., Hirohata, T., Hislop, T.G., et al. "Dietary Factors and Risk of Breast Cancer: Combined Analysis of 12 Case-Control Studies." *Journal of the National Cancer Institute* 82 (1990): 562-569.

Jacques, P.F., Chylack, L.T. "Epidemiologic Evidence of a Role for the Antioxidant Vitamins and Carotenoids in Cataract Prevention." *American Journal of Clinical Nutrition* 53 (1991): 352S-355S.

Knekt, P., Jarvinen, R., Seppanen, R., et al. "Dietary Antioxidants and the Risk of Lung Cancer." *American Journal of Epidemiology* 134 (1991): 471-479.

McLaughlin, J.K., Gridley, G., Block, G., et al. "Dietary Factors in Oral and Pharyngeal Cancer." *Journal of the National Cancer Institute* 80 (1988): 1237-1243.

Salonen, J.T., Salonen, R., Ihanainen, M., et al. "Blood Pressure, Dietary Fats, and Antioxidants." *American Journal of Clinical Nutrition* 48 (1988): 1226-1232.

Verreault, R., Chu, J., Mandelson, M., et al. "A Case-Control Study of Diet and Invasive Cervical Cancer." *International Journal of Cancer* 43 (1989): 1050-1054.

VITAMIN D

Chapuy, M.C., Arlot, M.E., Duboeuf, F., et al. "Vitamin D3 and Calcium to Prevent Hip Fractures in Elderly Women." *NEJM* 327 (1992): 1637-1642.

Dawson-Hughes, B., Dallal, G.E., Krall, E.A., et al. "Effect of Vitamin D Supplementation on Wintertime and Overall Bone Loss in Healthy Postmenopausal Women." *Annals of Internal Medicine* 115 (1991): 505-512.

Lips, P., van Ginkel, F.C., Jongen, M.J., et al. "Determinants of Vitamin D Status in Patients with Hip Fracture and in Elderly Control Subjects." *American Journal of Clinical Nutrition* 46 (1987): 1005-1010.

VITAMIN E

Blot, W.J., Li, J.Y., Taylor, P.R., et al. "Nutrition Intervention Trials in Linxian, China: Supplementation With Specific Vitamin/Mineral Combinations, Cancer Incidence, and Disease-Specific Mortality in the General Population." *Journal of the National Cancer Institute* 85 (1993): 1483-1492.

Gridley, G., McLaughlin, J.K., Block, G., et al. "Vitamin Supplement Use and Reduced Risk of Oral and Pharyngeal Cancer." *American Journal of Epidemiology* 135 (1992): 1083-1092.

Knekt, P., Aromaa, A., Maatela, J., et al. "Vitamin E and Cancer Prevention." *American Journal of Clinical Nutrition* 53 (1991): 283S-286S.

Knekt, P., Jarvinen, R., Seppanen, R., et al. "Dietary Antioxidants and the Risk of Lung Cancer." *American Journal of Epidemiology* 134 (1991): 471-479.

LeGardeur, B.Y., Lopez, S.A., Johnson, W.D. "A Case-Control Study of Serum Vitamins A, E, and C in Lung Cancer Patients." *Nutrition and Cancer* 14 (1990): 133-140.

Menkes, M.S., Comstock, G.W., Vuilleumier, J.P., et al. "Serum Beta-Carotene, Vitamins A and E, Selenium, and the Risk of Lung Cancer." *NEJM* 315 (1986): 1250-1254.

Meydani, S.N., Barklund, M.P., Liu, S., et al. "Vitamin E Supplementation Enhances Cell-Mediated Immunity in Healthy Elderly Subjects." *American Journal of Clinical Nutrition* 52 (1990): 557-563.

Palan, P.R., Mikhail, M.S., Basu, J., et al. "Plasma Levels of Antioxidant Beta-Carotene and Alpha-Tocopherol in Uterine Cervix Dysplasias and Cancer." *Nutrition and Cancer* 15 (1991): 13-20.

Rimm, E.B., Stampfer, M.J., Ascherio, A., et al. "Vitamin E Consumption and the Risk of Coronary Heart Disease in Men." *NEJM* 328 (1993): 1450-1456.

Stampfer, M.J., Hennekens, C.H., Manson, J.E., et al. "Vitamin E Consumption and the Risk of Coronary Heart Disease in Women." *NEJM* 328 (1993): 1444-1449.

Verreault, R., Chu, J., Mandelson, M., et al. "A Case-Control Study of Diet and Invasive Cervical Cancer." *International Journal of Cancer* 43 (1989): 1050-1054.

Wald, N.J., Boreham, J., Hayward, J.L., et al. "Plasma Retinol, Beta-Carotene, and Vitamin E Levels in Relation to the Future Risk of Breast Cancer." *British Journal of Cancer* 49 (1984): 321-324.

FOLIC ACID

Butterworth, C.E., Hatch, K.D., Macaluso, M., et al. "Folate Deficiency and Cervical Dysplasia." *JAMA* 367 (1992): 528-533.

Czeizel, A.E. "Prevention of Congenital Abnormalities by Periconceptional Multivitamin Supplementation." *British Medical Journal* 306 (1993): 1645-1648.

Czeizel, A.E., Dudas, I. "Prevention of the First Occurrence of Neural-Tube Defects by Periconceptional Vitamin Supplementation." *NEJM* 327 (1992): 1832-1835.

MRC Vitamin Study Research Group. "Prevention of Neural Tube Defects: Results of the Medical Research Council Vitamin Study." *Lancet* 338 (1991): 131-137.

Selhub, J., Jacques, P.F., Wilson, P.W., et al. "Vitamin Status and Intake as Primary Determinants of Homocysteinemia in an Elderly Population." *JAMA* 270 (1993): 2693-2698.

CALCIUM

Belizan, J.M., Villar, J., Pineda, O., et al. "Reduction of Blood Pressure with Calcium Supplementation in Young Adults." *JAMA* 249 (1983): 1161-1165.

Chapuy, M.C., Arlot, M.E., Duboeuf, F., et al. "Vitamin D3 and Calcium to Prevent Hip Fractures in Elderly Women." *NEJM* 327 (1992): 1637-1642.

Dawson-Hughes, B., Dallal, G.E., Krali, E.A., et al. "A Controlled Trial of the Effect of Calcium Supplementation on Bone Density in Postmenopausal Women." *NEJM* 323 (1990): 878-883.

Garland, C., Barrett-Connor, E., Rossof, A.H., et al. "Dietary Vitamin D and Calcium and Risk of Colorectal Cancer: A 19-Year Prospective Study in Men." *Lancet* 1 (1985): 307-309.

Grobbee, D.E., Hofman, A. "Effect of Calcium Supplementation on Diastolic Blood Pressure in Young People with Mild Hypertension." *Lancet* 2 (1986): 703-707.

Harlan, W.R., Hull, A.L., Schmouder, R.L., et al. "Blood Pressure and Nutrition in Adults: The National Health and Nutrition Examination Survey." *American Journal of Epidemiology* 120 (1984): 17-28.

Johnston, C.C., Miller, J.Z., Slemenda, C.W., et al. "Calcium Supplementation and Increases in Bone Mineral Density in Children." *NEJM* 327 (1992): 82-87.

Lloyd, T., Andon, M.B., Rollings, N., et al. "Calcium Supplementation and Bone Mineral Density in Adolescent Girls." *JAMA* 270 (1993): 841-844.

IRON

Salonen, J.T., Nyyssonen, K., Korpela, H., et al. "High Stored Iron Levels Are Associated With Excess Risk of Myocardial Infarction In Eastern Finnish Men." *Circulation* 86 (1992): 803-811.

Sempos, C.T., Looker, A.C., Gillum, R.F., et al. "Body Iron Stores and the Risk of Coronary Heart Disease." *NEJM* 330 (1994): 1119-1124.

MAGNESIUM

Ascherio, A., Rimm, E.B., Giovannucci, E.L., et al. "A Prospective Study of Nutritional Factors and Hypertension Among US Men." *Circulation* 86 (1992): 1475-1484.

Joffres, M.R., Reed, D.M., Yano, K. "Relationship of Magnesium Intake and Other Dietary Factors to Blood Pressure: The Honolulu Heart Study." *American Journal of Clinical Nutrition* 45 (1987): 469-475.

Lind, L., Lithell, H., Pollare, T., et al. "Blood Pressure Response During Long-Term Treatment with Magnesium Is Dependent on Magnesium Status: A Double-Blind, Placebo-Controlled Study in Essential Hypertension and in Subjects with High-Normal Blood Pressure." *American Journal of Hypertension* 4 (1991): 674-679.

Motoyama, T., Sano, H., Suzuki, H., et al. "Oral Magnesium Treatment and Sodium Pump in Patients with Essential Hypertension." (abst) *Circulation* 74 (1986) supp. 2, 329.

Widman, L., Wester, P.O., Stegmayr, B.K., et al. "The Dose-Dependent Reduction in Blood Pressure Through Administration of Magnesium: A Double Blind Placebo Controlled Cross-Over Study." *American Journal of Hypertension* 6 (1993): 41-45.

SELENIUM

Beaglehole, R., Jackson, R., Watkinson, J., et al. "Decreased Blood Selenium and Risk of Myocardial Infarction." *International Journal of Epidemiology* 19 (1990): 918-922.

Blot, W.J., Li, J.Y., Taylor, P.R., et al. "Nutrition Intervention Trials in Linxian, China: Supplementation With Specific Vitamin/Mineral Combinations, Cancer Incidence, and Disease-Specific Mortality in the General Population." *Journal of the National Cancer Institute* 85 (1993): 1483-1492.

Hunter, D.J., Morris, J.S., Stampfer, M.J., et al. "A Prospective Study of Selenium Status and Breast Cancer Risk." *JAMA* 264 (1990): 1128-1131.

Moore, J.A., Noiva, R., Wells, I.C. "Selenium Concentrations in Plasma of Patients with Arteriographically Defined Coronary Atherosclerosis." *Clinical Chemistry* 30 (1984): 1171-1173.

Salonen, J.T., Alfthan, G., Huttunen, J.K., et al. "Association Between Serum Selenium and the Risk of Cancer." *American Journal of Epidemiology* 120 (1984): 342-349.

Salonen, J.T., Alfthan, G., Pikkarainen, J., et al. "Association Between Cardiovascular Death and Myocardial Infarction and Serum Selenium in a Matched-Pair Longitudinal Study." *Lancet* 2 (1982): 175-179.

Salonen, J.T., Salonen, R., Lappetelainen, R., et al. "Risk of Cancer in Relation to Serum Concentrations of Selenium and Vitamins A and E: Matched Case-Control Analysis of Prospective Data." *British Medical Journal* 290 (1985): 417-420.

van der Brandt, P.A., Goldbohm, R.A., van't Veer, P., et al. "A Prospective Cohort Study on Toenail Selenium Levels and Risk of Gastrointestinal Cancer." *Journal of the National Cancer Institute* 85 (1993): 224-229.

Willett, W.C., Polk, B.F., Morris, J.S., et al. "Prediagnostic Serum Selenium and Risk of Cancer." *Lancet* 2 (1983): 130-134.

ZINC

Castillo-Duran, C., Heresi, G., Fisberg, M., Uauy, R. "Controlled Trial of Zinc Supplementation During Recovery from Malnutrition: Effects on Growth and Immune Function." *American Journal of Clinical Nutrition* 45 (1987): 602-608.

Duchateau, J., Delespesse, G., Vereecke, P. "Influence of Oral Zinc Supplementation on the Lymphocyte Response to Mitogens of Normal Subjects." *American Journal of Clinical Nutrition* 34 (1981): 88-93

Duchateau, J., Delepresse, G., Vrijens, R., et al. "Beneficial Effects of Oral Zinc Supplementation on the Immune Response of Old People." *American Journal of Medicine* 70 (1981): 1001-1004.

INDEX

NOTES:

About the Authors

Dr. Art Ulene has been known to television viewers over the past two decades through his medical reports on the NBC "Today Show" and the ABC "HOME Show." Additionally, he is the author of numerous books and the producer of several video and audio programs. He lives in Los Angeles.

Dr. Ulene's co-author is his daughter, Dr. Val Ulene, also a medical doctor. In addition to the medical degree which she received from Columbia University, Dr. Val Ulene holds a master's degree in public health. She lives in New York City.